CERRITOS COLLEGE LIBRARY
Norwalk, California
DISCARD

JAN 4 2008

Lukan's Documentation for Physical Therapist Assistants

THIRD EDITION

D1119794

THIRD EDITION

Lukan's Documentation for Physical Therapist Assistants

Wendy D. Bircher, PT, EdD

Director/Associate Professor
Physical Therapist Assistant Program
San Juan College
Farmington, New Mexico

F. A. DAVIS COMPANY · Philadelphia

RM 705 .L84 2008
Bircher, Wendy D.
Lukan's documentation for
physical therapist

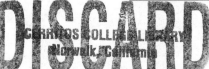

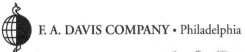

DISCARD
CERRITOS COLLEGE LIBRARY
Norwalk, California

F. A. Davis Company
1915 Arch Street
Philadelphia, PA 19103
www.fadavis.com

Copyright © 2008 by F. A. Davis Company

Copyright © 2007 by F. A. Davis Company. All rights reserved. This product is protected by copyright. No part of it may be reproduced, stored in a retrieval system, or transmitted in any form or by any means, electronic, mechanical, photocopying, recording, or otherwise, without written permission from the publisher.

Printed in the United States of America

Last digit indicates print number: 10 9 8 7 6 5 4 3 2 1

Publisher: Margaret Biblis
Acquisitions Editor: Melissa A. Duffield
Developmental Editor: Yvonne Gillam
Manager of Content Development: Deborah J. Thorp
Art and Design Manager: Carolyn O'Brien

As new scientific information becomes available through basic and clinical research, recommended treatments and drug therapies undergo changes. The author and publisher have done everything possible to make this book accurate, up to date, and in accord with accepted standards at the time of publication. The author, editors, and publisher are not responsible for errors or omissions or for consequences from application of the book, and make no warranty, expressed or implied, in regard to the contents of the book. Any practice described in this book should be applied by the reader in accordance with professional standards of care used in regard to the unique circumstances that may apply in each situation. The reader is advised always to check product information (package inserts) for changes and new information regarding dose and contraindications before administering any drug. Caution is especially urged when using new or infrequently ordered drugs.

Library of Congress Cataloging-in-Publication Data
Bircher, Wendy D.
   Lukan's documentation for physical therapist assistants/Wendy D.
Bircher. — 3rd ed.
      p. ; cm.
   Rev. ed. of: Documentation for physical therapist assistants /
Marianne Lukan. 2nd ed. c2001.
   Includes bibliographical references and index.
   ISBN-13: 978-0-8036-1709-4
   ISBN-10: 0-8036-1709-7
 1. Physical therapy assistants. 2. Physical therapy—Documentation.
3. Medical records. I. Lukan, Marianne, 1940- II. Lukan, Marianne,
1940-. Documentation for physical therapist assistants. III. Title. IV.
Title: Documentation for physical therapist assistants.
   [DNLM: 1. Forms and Records Control—methods. 2. Physical Therapy
(Specialty)—organization & administration. 3. Allied Health
Personnel. 4. Medical Records—standards. WB 460 B617L 2008]
   RM705. L 84 2008
   615. 8′2—dc22
                                                              2007024657

Authorization to photocopy items for internal or personal use, or the internal or personal use of specific clients, is granted by F. A. Davis Company for users registered with the Copyright Clearance Center (CCC) Transactional Reporting Service, provided that the fee of $.10 per copy is paid directly to CCC, 222 Rosewood Drive, Danvers, MA 01923. For those organizations that have been granted a photocopy license by CCC, a separate system of payment has been arranged. The fee code for users of the Transactional Reporting Service is:8036-1709/08 + $.10.

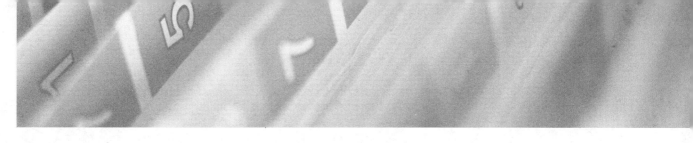

Preface

As a physical therapist and teacher for 30 years, I have found many textbooks that have given educational support to students while providing additional instructional support to teachers. These textbooks cover many subjects by providing information students need to learn for specific skills in their related field of study. The requests from students and instructors continue for a documentation textbook that will teach the student the necessary steps required for proper documentation and will assist the student in producing such documentation related to patient care and treatment.

In addition, with the advent of computerized documentation and access to the Internet, it is important to provide the student with additional examples of forms used in various types of facilities and additional examples of documentation types and to provide access for instructors to different websites for support. It is the hope of this author that the third edition of this documentation textbook will provide the student with the information and material necessary to become a good therapist who can provide appropriate and billable comments in documentation related to patient care and treatment.

GUIDE TO PHYSICAL THERAPIST PRACTICE

Some of the information in this edition includes guidelines from the second edition of the *Guide to Physical Therapist Practice,* a reference published by the American Physical Therapy Association. Information included in the *Guide* provides the student with guidelines for ethical practice, guidelines for documentation, and examples of documentation templates. The *Guide* remains a necessary resource for all physical therapists and physical therapist assistants practicing in today's clinical setting.

EXPANSION OF CHAPTERS

This edition expands several chapters and adds information related to the responsibility of documentation for the physical therapist assistant in a clinical setting, importance of documentation, steps involved in proper documentation, use of the SOAP note format, relationship of documentation to patient issues, importance of documentation in legal settings, and review of documentation requirements to prepare for the national licensing examination.

ADDITIONAL PRACTICE EXERCISES

In response to the demand for more exercises, more practice exercises have been added to all chapters, and it is the hope of this author that these supplementary exercises will provide the student with the means to address documentation in various clinical settings. It is also hoped that the student will have an increased understanding of the importance of, and the information included in, each section of the SOAP note.

—Wendy Bircher

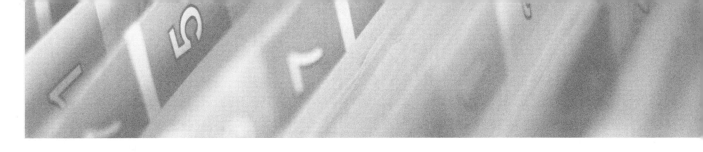

Reviewers

KENNETH R. AMSLER, PhD, PT
Chair, Program Director
South University
Palm Beach Gardens, Florida

LINDA CLARKSON, BA, PTA
ACCE
Kansas City Kansas Community College
Kansas City, Kansas

KAREN COUPE, PT, DPT, MEd
Faculty
Keiser College
Ft. Lauderdale, Florida

DEBORAH R. EVANS
Instructor, PTA Program
Stark State College
Louisville, Ohio

WANDA GATTSHALL-PERESIC, PT, DPT, MS
Coordinator, PTA Program
Kansas City Kansas Community College
Kansas City, Kansas

CHRISTINE KOWALSKI, EdD, PTA
Chair, Health Sciences Department
Montana State University, Great Falls-College
of Technology
Great Falls, Montana

PENELOPE LESCHER, PT, MA, MCSP
Former Director, PTA Program
Chesapeake Area Consortium
Hollidaysburg, Pennsylvania

MARLENE MEDIN, PT, MEd
Director, PTA Program
Linn State Technical College
Jefferson City, Missouri

JOHN MILLER, Jr, PTA, BS
Assistant Professor
Baltimore City Community College
Baltimore, Maryland

THERESE MILLIS, BSPT
Instructor, PTA Program
Arapahoe Community College
Littleton, Colorado

JOANNA W. NICHOLSON, MA, PTA
Instructor
Central Piedmont Community College
Charlotte, North Carolina

STEFANIE D. PALMA, PT, DPT, MEd
Faculty
Georgia State University
Atlanta, Georgia

CAROL G. PLISNER, PT
Coordinator, PTA Program
Macomb Community College
Clinton Township, Michigan

KIM SNYDER, PTA, MEd
Coordinator, PTA Program
Southwestern Illinois College
Belleville, Illinois

VICKY TROST, PT, DPT
Director, PTA Program, and ACCE
Clarkson College
Omaha, Nebraska

MARTHA ZIMMERMAN, PT, MA
Director, PTA Program
Caldwell Community College and Technical
Institute
Hudson, North Carolina

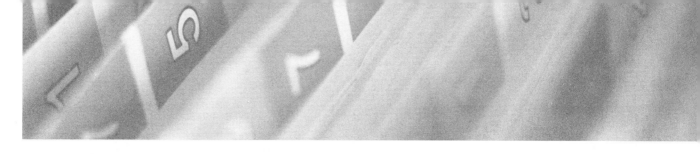

Acknowledgments

I would like to thank all of my students who made this quest necessary with their continuous questions related to documentation. I would like to thank my fellow faculty members Amy Cooper, Sonja Lawrence, and Therese Millis for their unending support and input for the revision of this textbook. In addition, I would like to thank Margaret Bilbis, Melissa Duffield, and Yvonne Gillam from F. A. Davis for their vision and willingness to place such an important undertaking in my hands. Last, but not least, I would like to thank my husband, John, and my son, Matthew, for always being there and helping me move forward with my life choices.

Contents

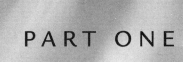

PART ONE

Why Is Documentation Important?

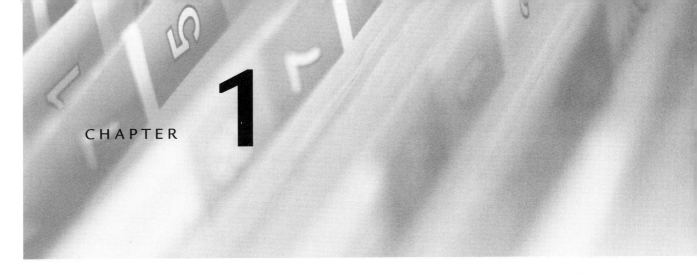

CHAPTER 1

Introduction to Documentation

LEARNING OBJECTIVES

After studying this chapter, the student will be able to:

☐ Define documentation.

☐ Identify the significance of documentation in patient care.

☐ Describe the differences between the Nagi Disablement Model and International Classification of Functioning (ICF) classifications for documentation.

☐ Describe changes in referral for physical therapy that have occurred since the early 1960s.

☐ Explain how changes in referral for physical therapy affected the evolution of responsibilities of the Physical Therapist (PT) and Physical Therapist Assistant (PTA).

☐ Identify the major factor that currently influences the provision of health-care services and the responsibilities of the PT and PTA.

☐ Describe the role of documentation in patient care.

☐ Discuss how documentation benefits the PT and PTA professions and the patient.

INTRODUCTION

Having been introduced to documentation over 25 years ago, I have witnessed the changes that have occurred to ensure proper patient care, documentation, and reimbursement for that care. With the introduction of physical therapist assistants (PTAs), some of the documentation responsibilities have shifted to the PTA. The PTA now bears as much responsibility for proper documentation as does the physical therapist (PT).

This book discusses the documentation tasks expected from the PTA, the importance of quality documentation, and the best way to produce thorough and proper documentation that fills the needs of the patient, the facility, and third-party payers and that addresses the legal and ethical issues that surround quality patient care.

DOCUMENTATION AND ITS SIGNIFICANCE

Webster's dictionary defines *document* as "anything written that gives information or supplies evidence." *Documentation* is defined as "the assembling of documents, the using of documentary evidence to support original written work, or the evidence itself ... , the classifying and making available of knowledge as a procedure."[1]

Evidence of Patient Care

In any health-care facility, service is provided to the patient by more than one medical professional. Records or medical charts are kept to document the treatments given, services performed, and services to be provided. Medical charts provide information that authenticates the care given to the patient and the reasons for providing that care. Thus, documentation is written so legal proof exists that medical care was given to the patient, and this evidence is available for future use. If the treatment provided is not documented in the chart, it is assumed the treatment was not provided. "If it isn't written, it didn't happen" is a good rule.

Accountability for Patient Care

The written record is the mechanism through which the health-care professional is held accountable for the medical care provided to the patient. The record is reviewed by the third-party payer to determine the reimbursement value of the medical services, and the information is studied to measure or determine the efficacy of the treatment procedures. The reader of the medical record finds the rationale that supports the medical necessity for the treatment, the activities involved in that treatment process, and the legal basis for such treatment.

Importance of Documentation

The impact of poorly written physical therapy documentation is illustrated by the following story based on a true experience of a PT in 1998. The situation includes some of the topics and information discussed in this textbook. However, in some instances, the situation only alludes to this information. A practice exercise at the end of the chapter challenges you to identify these topics.

The Experience

A PT, who worked for a home health-care agency, was contacted by an attorney for the prosecution in a child abuse case that involved a patient who had previously been under her care. The father had been accused of shaking his son violently enough to cause brain damage. The child was last seen by the therapist more than 3 years ago. Additionally, the therapist received a phone call from the PTA who had also worked with this patient under the PT's supervision.

The PTA informed the PT that she was being called to testify by the attorney for the defense, not for the prosecution, in the same court case. The PTA was worried about the case and having to testify for the first time in a federal court. Because the PT had supervised the PTA during this time, how could they present their information from opposite sides? Needless to say, both individuals were concerned about the legality of testifying against each other, especially because the PT had supervised the PTA in the care of this patient. Because 3 years had passed since this patient had received treatment, the PT hoped that the records regarding the patient's treatment were complete enough to ensure that the patient had received appropriate therapeutic intervention from the therapists and had correctly documented the role of the father in his son's injury (shaken baby syndrome) and his son's subsequent recovery.

The PT and PTA met with the attorneys for each side separately. They each reviewed the medical chart from the hospital that the child had been admitted to following the incident in question and the records completed by the PT and PTA while working for the home health-care agency. The patient had been an 8-month-old infant when the father became angry about his crying. In an attempt to get the baby to be quiet, he had "shaken" the baby violently causing damage to the frontal and occipital lobes. It was reported that the father knew he had caused severe damage to his son and had immediately brought him to the emergency room at a nearby hospital. The mother had been contacted at work and had arrived in the emergency room just as her husband was being arrested for child abuse. The child initially presented with right-sided paralysis, visual impairment, and increased muscle tone.

After being treated for 2 years, the patient had completely regained normal function in all areas of development and normal vision was restored. The defense was attempting to keep the father out of jail and return him to his family. They felt he had paid for his mistake by realizing what he had done to his son. He followed all the guidelines of the court, which included attending therapy sessions when he was not in jail and spending supervised time with his son. There had been no further incidents of abuse, and the baby appeared to have an excellent relationship with his father. The prosecution wanted the father to continue with his incarceration and, because he was considered a child abuser, not to be allowed to see his son upon his release.

The PT reviewed her notes with the prosecuting attorney (Fig. 1–1). The PT's notes were two to three lines, at most, which was all that had been required by the home health-care agency, at that time. The PTA's notes were fairly complete and appeared to follow the PT's plan of care. However, the progress notes certainly wouldn't meet the present criteria for third-party payers such as Medicaid or Medicare! How were the PT and PTA going to respond to cross-examination by the opposing lawyers when their notes simply stated "pt. is improving" and "pt. tolerated treatment well"? These notes did not help either therapist recall the specifics of the patient's physical therapy treatment sessions about which they needed to testify. Both individuals wished their notes had been written more clearly and with more specific goals and outcomes!

2-8-98: Pt. feeling better today. Pt. was seen for a 30 minute therapy visit.
       S: Mom told PTA that her son is cranky and stiff.
       O: Worked on sitting and rolling.
       A: Pt. able to sit by himself for short time periods.
       P: Continue PT sessions.

Figure 1—1 A note from the medical chart containing the physical therapy progress notes for the patient written in 1998.

The notes were reviewed, the information was recalled, and the PT and PTA were ready to testify. During their trips home, both the PT and PTA realized how necessary it was to provide quality documentation and found that the statement, "if it isn't written, it didn't happen" took on more meaning. This court experience would have been so much easier for both therapists if the written notes had been in the same format currently required by third-party payers (discussed in Chapter 3). To see the difference between 1998 and 2006 standards of care, compare the example of a note included in the court testimony (Fig. 1–1) with the example of how the session would have been documented today (Fig. 1–2). (Definitions of the abbreviations used in the notes are in Appendix A.)

EVOLUTION OF PT AND PTA RESPONSIBILITIES AND THE ROLE OF DOCUMENTATION

The preceding 1998 versus 2006 event is an example of how documentation has evolved over time. This evolution has been a result of the changing responsibilities of the PT and PTA for treatment and documentation.

The Past

Three events have influenced the evolution of PT and PTA responsibilities and the role of documentation in patient care. These three events are changes in physicians' referrals for physical therapy, the enactment of Medicare, and the development of documentation classifications.

Changes in Physicians' Referrals for Physical Therapy

The method by which physicians prescribe physical therapy has changed throughout the profession's short history. The changes have increased the PT's clinical decision-making power, led to the development of the physical therapy diagnosis, and offered the opportunity for autonomy in the practice of therapy.

2-8-06: Pt. has been seen at home for 10 physical therapy visits since hospital d/c on 1-5-2006. The physical therapy evaluation was on 1-8-06 and visits were set for 2x/week by the PTA and supervisory visits with the PT once a month. The session today was for 45 minutes. Pt. currently functions at a 6-7 month level in gross motor skills for his chronological age of 10.5 months. Mother reports central vision is still impaired as the pt. continues to turn his head and use his peripheral vision. The pt. will be seen for six more visits before re-evaluation and re-certification.

S: Mother stated the patient is not sleeping through the night and becomes quite agitated until she swaddles him and rocks him for several hours. Pt. continues to exhibit moderate hypertonicity overall with the right side more involved. Mother questions her son's development and is concerned about her husband who is unable to come home.

O: Patient can sit independently when placed in a sitting position, for over 1 minute. He can roll independently from prone to supine and supine to prone without using tone and with an appropriate flexor pattern. Patient can maintain an independent prone position on extended forearms for over 30 seconds and is beginning to pull his hips into flexion to approximate a four-point crawl position when in a prone position. Patient's PROM and AROM remain WNL and strength is 4/5 overall. Pt.'s alignment remains symmetrical and protective responses are present in all positions and all directions with a minimal delay noted on the right side. Independent manual muscle testing remains inappropriate due to the patient's young age. Exercises included positioning in independent sit, prone and side sit with transitions in and out of each position. Transitions are accomplished with minimal assist.

A: Improvement in patient's gross motor skills continues with a good potential to meet the goal of independent sit with transition from the floor to sit within the next month. Hypertonicity has decreased from moderate to mild overall and patient is beginning to increase flexor patterns for improved sitting balance with an anterior pelvic tilt and beginning four-point crawl positioning. The home exercise program was reviewed with the mother and she correctly performed a return demonstration of all activities.

P: Patient is scheduled 2x/week for 2 weeks with the PTA monitoring the home exercise program and gross motor progress and mother's handling skills. Programming will focus on increasing independent transition from floor to sit and independent four-point crawl position held for 30 seconds by the end of the next session. The PTA will set the supervisory visit with PT for 2-12-06.

_____ Joan Therapist, LPTA
PT Lic. #123

Figure 1—2   An example of how the note from 1998 could be rewritten to meet the requirements for a note written in 2006.

THE PHYSICAL THERAPY PRESCRIPTION.   Until the early 1960s, a patient commonly came to a PT with a referral from a physician in the form of a physical therapy prescription. That is, it read much like a medication prescription, as illustrated in Figure 1–3, or the instructions were more general, such as ultrasound, massage, or exercise. The PT was required to follow the physician's orders and provide the treatment as prescribed. If the PT did not agree with the treatment plan, he or she needed to discuss this with the physician in an attempt to agree on a more appropriate treatment plan. The PT was not always successful in convincing the physician to change the order; thus, the physical therapy treatment provided may not have

P. T. Knowes, M.D.
123 Medical Building, Suite 1
Yourtown, NM 87405
(505) 111-222

Physical Therapy for Hazel Jones:

US at 1.5 w/cm2 for 5 min. to the right deltoid insertion, followed by 10 min. of massage. AAROM 10 rep. for abduction (not to exceed 165°), flexion (not to exceed 170°), and external rotation (not to exceed 25°).

P. T. Knowes, MD

Figure 1—3   Illustration of a physician's order for physical therapy that tells the physical therapist exactly what to do. It resembles a medication prescription.

been as appropriate or effective as possible. The PT was practicing at the level of a technician, following precise directions from the physician, and documenting briefly that the treatment was provided and whether the patient was improving. Autonomy in practice was not evident.

EVALUATE AND TREAT.   In the early 1960s, PTs began convincing some physicians that a PT had the training and knowledge to evaluate a patient's neuromusculoskeletal system and determine the treatment appropriate for the patient's condition. A patient brought a referral from the physician that provided the diagnosis and stated "evaluate and treat." The responsibilities of the PT expanded to include (1) determining the physical therapy diagnosis on the basis of evaluation results and (2) defining the interventions or treatment plan. The physical therapy problem would be described in terms of the neuromusculoskeletal abnormality, and the treatment plan would be directed toward correcting or minimizing this problem. The PT needed evaluation skills to identify physical therapy problems and to make clinical decisions regarding treatment of those problems. Writing the initial, interim, and discharge evaluations became additional documentation responsibilities for every PT.

The first academic program for training the PTA was established in 1967. The PTA assumed the role as the technician providing the physical therapy treatments under the direct guidance and supervision of the PT. Writing progress notes was a documentation responsibility shared by the PT and PTA.

DIRECT ACCESS.   Direct access allows a person access to the medical care system directly through a PT, without a physician's referral. The PT may evaluate the patient to determine whether the patient's condition is a disorder treatable by physical therapy. Nebraska has allowed direct access since 1957. California eliminated the need for a physician's referral in 1968. When Maryland's Physical Therapy Practice Act was amended in 1979 to allow direct access, many American Physical Therapy Association (APTA) state chapters launched their amendment campaigns. Today, the few states that do not have direct-access language in their state practice acts[2] do have direct-access legislation in progress.

Direct access gives the PT opportunity for autonomy, but it also requires the PT to have the skills and knowledge to recognize conditions that are not problems that can be helped by physical therapy. The PT is responsible for referring a patient to a physician or other appropriate health-care provider when the patient exhibits signs and symptoms of a systemic disorder or a problem that is beyond the scope of practice or expertise of the PT. The PTA is responsible for reporting any sign or symptom or lack of progress that indicates a need for the PT to reevaluate the patient. For more information about direct access and the states that currently have direct access, go to this website: www.apta.org (Once you have accessed the website, click on advocacy, state government affairs, and finally, resources for chapters.).

The focus of a PT's education has had to change, increasing the emphasis on scientific knowledge, evaluation skills, critical thinking, and research and decreasing the emphasis on treatment skills. A PTA's training, although still focusing on treatment skills, has expanded to emphasize the theories behind these treatment skills. This expansion provides the PTA with the knowledge to make clinical decisions within the parameters of the PT's treatment plan and the PTA's level of training and scope of practice. For example, in home health settings, the PTA's responsibilities have evolved to allow the PTA to treat patients when the PT is not on the premises but is accessible through telecommunications. These parameters vary and are set by the individual states in which the PTA practices.

Establishment of Medicare

Before 1970, documentation in the medical chart was not always thorough or specific. Health-care providers knew documentation should be done well, but unfortunately, poor-quality documentation was easy to find. Typically, progress notes were brief, consisting of one or two lines, and were subjective and/or judgmental in nature. For example: "Patient feeling better today" (see Fig. 1–1). No standards for documentation existed, and those paying the health-care bills did not demand accountability for those bills.

In the mid-1960s, this changed when the Health Insurance for the Aged and Disabled Act, known as Medicare, was enacted. Thus, the federal government began purchasing medical care for the elderly. Within the Department of Health and Human Services, the Health Care Financing Administration issued standards for documentation to be followed for all patients receiving Medicare. Other insurance companies soon followed Medicare's example. Those paying the medical bills demanded that health-care providers be held accountable for the dollars spent. This accountability was determined through proper documentation that clearly identified the physical therapy problem, treatment goals and plans, and treatment results.[3]

Comparison of Documentation Classifications

Several taxonomies have been developed to aid in the documentation process for physical therapy services. Nagi's Model of Disablement[4] of 1969 was used as the groundwork to help revise the World Health Organization's *International Classification of Impairments, Disabilities, and Handicaps*[5] (ICIDH) in 1980 and the *International Classification of Functioning, Disability, and Health*[6] (ICF) in 2001. Additionally, in 1992, The National Center for Medical Rehabilitation Research (NCMRR) provided support for specific definitions related to disability.[7] Specifically, these classification methods help provide common language in the care of the disabled patient. A summary of the classifications can be found in Table 1–1.

These taxonomies developed a common definition for the following terms used in documentation:

Impairment: A loss or abnormality of a physiological, psychological, or anatomical structure or function

Functional limitation: A restriction of the ability to perform an activity or a task in an efficient, typically expected, or competent manner

Disability: An inability to perform or a limitation in the performance of actions, tasks, and activities usually expected in specific social roles and physical environments

FUNCTION VERSUS IMPAIRMENT. For proper documentation to occur in the therapy field, function and impairment must be differentiated. According to the preceding classifications, an impairment can lead to a functional problem, whereas a functional problem may not always cause an impairment. A functional problem is usually patient-specific.

The Present

Our health-care system is now in a state of transition; services provided to patients are being reduced because of limited financial resources. The physical therapy provider is placed in a position of competing for these limited funds. Physical therapy services will not be reimbursed when the treatments are not effective and efficient. The patient or client seeks physical therapy because of problems resulting from a disease or injury that prevents the person from functioning in his or her environment. Therapeutic interventions are directed toward

Table 1-1 Documentation Classification Methods		
Definition and use of the ICIDH and ICF classifications	**Definition and use of the Nagi Disablement Model**	**National Center for Medical Rehabilitation Research Definition of Disabilities[7]**
ICIDH Classification: Provided a uniform standard of language for the description of health and health-related issues (1980).[5] ICF Classification: Updated the ICIDH classification to integrate the biomedical, psychological, and social aspects of diseases and their related disabilities, handicaps, and impairments (2001).[6]	Nagi's Disablement Model: Model of disablement to correlate impairment and functional limitations (1969).[4] This model provided a definitive summary of an active pathology with the relationship to the resulting impairment, functional limitation, and disability.	National Center for Medical Rehabilitation Research (NCMRR) Definition of Disabilities:[7] Provides a description of services to patients with impairments, functional limitations and disabilities, or changes in the status of these areas as a result of injury, disease, or other causes related to the pathology and societal limitations they might affect.

improving or restoring the patient's functional abilities by minimizing or resolving these problems in the most cost-effective manner.

Documentation that meets today's standards provides the basis for research to measure functional outcomes and identify the most effective and efficient treatment procedures. Documentation must describe what functional activities the patient has difficulty performing and must show how the interventions are effective in improving or restoring the patient's function. Documentation must be done properly if PTs and PTAs are to survive financially. Without proper documentation for the specific treatment given to a patient, reimbursement will not occur.

ROLE OF DOCUMENTATION IN PATIENT CARE

Three themes are repeated in this text:

1. Documentation records the quality of and the ability to replicate the patient's care.
2. Documentation constructs a legal report of patient care.
3. Documentation provides the basis for reimbursement for patient care.

A Record of the Quality of Patient Care

The term quality care as used in this text refers to medical care that is appropriate for and focused on the patient's problems relevant to the diagnosis. Quality physical therapy care is defined as care that follows the *Standards of Practice* for physical therapy published by the APTA.[8]

To provide high-quality medical care, good communication among health-care professionals is absolutely essential. The PTA must accurately and consistently communicate with the supervising PT. The PTA may also share and coordinate information with other medical providers, including other PTs and PTAs who may fill in when the PTA is absent, occupational therapists (OTs), and occupational therapy assistants, nurses and nursing assistants, physicians and physician assistants, speech pathologists, psychologists, social workers, and chaplains. The medical record is the avenue through which the medical team communicates regarding:

■ Identification of the patient's problems
■ Solutions for the patient's problems
■ Plans for the patient's discharge
■ Coordination of the continuum of care

This communication process helps ensure the quality of care.

The quality of care provided by the medical facility is determined by a review of the existing records. This review process is a way to monitor and influence the quality of health care provided by the facility. The information in the medical record is reviewed or audited for three purposes:

1. *Quality assurance.* Records are reviewed to determine whether the health care provided meets legal standards and appropriate health-care criteria. This is done externally by agencies accrediting the facility and internally by a quality-assurance committee. Problem areas are identified and plans are made for correction and improvement. This is a continuous process; the quality-assurance committee usually meets on a regular basis, and accrediting agencies audit a facility every few years. PTAs are permitted to serve on the quality-assurance committee.
2. *Research and education.* Information in the medical record is used for research and for student instruction. Research helps validate treatment techniques and identify new and better ways to provide health care. The record is used for retrospective studies that measure outcomes to determine the most cost-effective treatment approach to patient care. Students are encouraged to question and challenge the treatment procedures as part of their learning process.
3. *Reimbursement.* Third-party payers, such as insurance companies and Medicare, decide how to reimburse for medical care by reading the documentation in the medical record. The record must show that the patient's problems were identified and that treatment was directed toward solving those problems and discharging the patient.

Documentation
Standards and Criteria

Documentation that ensures quality care follows the standards and criteria set by a variety of sources. Although the standards are similar, the PTA should be familiar with the criteria required by:

- The federal government
- State governments
- Professional associations
- Accrediting agencies
- Health-care facilities

FEDERAL GOVERNMENT.   The federal government funds and administers Medicare (a type of medical insurance coverage for the elderly). The PTA must follow Medicare documentation requirements when treating a patient with this type of insurance. Because these requirements change frequently and can become complicated, the PTA must stay informed and up-to-date in his or her knowledge of Medicare requirements. For more information, go to this website: www.cms.hhs.gov[9]

STATE GOVERNMENTS.   Although funded by the federal government, Medicaid, a government program providing health care to the poor, is administered by the individual state governments. State governments also fund medical assistance and workers' compensation programs that have specific documentation criteria for patients with these types of insurance. The state may ask that specific data from the medical record be reported annually. Other documentation criteria determined at the state level may be influenced by the state's physical therapy legislation. The PTA must be well informed about the rules, regulations, and guidelines of the Physical Therapy Practice Act in the state where he or she wishes to practice.

PROFESSIONAL ASSOCIATIONS.   Associations can recommend documentation standards, such as the APTA's *Guidelines for Physical Therapy Documentation.*[10] These standards are the basis for the documentation instructions in this textbook and can be found in Appendix D.

ACCREDITING AGENCIES.   Accrediting agencies provide standards that health-care facilities must follow to meet accreditation criteria, including documentation requirements. Hospitals are accredited by the Joint Commission on Accreditation of Healthcare Organizations (JCAHO).[11] Rehabilitation facilities are accredited by the Commission on Accreditation of Rehabilitation Facilities (CARF).[12] PT and PTA educational programs also receive accreditation through the Commission on Accreditation for Physical Therapy Education (CAPTE) that introduces the concept of accreditation to students in PT and PTA programs.[13]

HEALTH-CARE FACILITIES.   Each health-care facility has its own documentation criteria; most facilities incorporate federal, state, and professional standards into their own procedures. The PTA can follow all standards and criteria by remembering this good rule: You can follow the policies and procedures of the facility where you work if they do not place you in a situation that is outside the scope of practice for your field or in a situation where the therapeutic intervention is inappropriate or unethical.

SUMMARY   Documenting in the medical record is one of the many responsibilities of the PTA. The medical record is a legal document that proves that medical care was given and holds the health-care providers accountable for the quality of the care given. It is an avenue for constant communication among health-care providers that enables identification of goals and monitoring of treatment progress. Insurance representatives read the medical record to determine whether to reimburse for the medical services provided. Historically, the PT was a technician, providing physical therapy treatments that were prescribed, in detail, by the physician. Responsibilities have evolved such that the PT is now an evaluator, consultant, manager, and practitioner seeing patients (clients) without a physician's referral. The PTA provides treatment under the guidance and supervision of the PT.

Physical therapy services must be provided in an efficient and cost-effective manner because financial resources to fund health care are no longer as easily accessible. The

---

Box 1-1   Implications For the PTA

Legal Issues

The medical record, and all that is contained within it, comprises a legal document and legal proof of the quality of care provided. The record protects the patient and the health-care providers should any questions arise in the future regarding the patient's care. Health-care providers work under the constant shadow of a possible malpractice lawsuit for each patient for which they come into contact. Months or years after a patient received treatment, the patient can become dissatisfied, leading to questions about the medical care received. Often these questions result in lawsuits, and many cases go to court because of the patient's claim that injury or illness was caused by an accident or negligence on the part of someone else. The PT, and possibly the PTA, may be called to testify in court about the therapy provided to the patient. Clear and accurate documentation is the best defense, demonstrating that safe and thorough patient care was provided.

Reimbursement Issues

The insurance company or organization paying for the patient's medical services determines the reimbursement rate from the information recorded in the medical chart. Payment is often denied when the documentation does not clearly provide the rationale to support the medical care provided. With some insurance plans, the caregiver must provide effective patient care while containing the costs within a preset payment amount. The caregiver demonstrates accountability for these costs by thoroughly and properly documenting the care provided.

---

outcomes now must focus on improving the client's **functional** abilities. Research must be done to measure the outcomes or results of physical therapy procedures and to define the most effective and efficient treatments for accomplishing the functional goals. Proper documentation facilitates this research.

The provision of up-to-date and valid physical therapy services will be ensured through documentation that meets the standards and criteria set by the federal and the state governments, professional agencies, accrediting agencies, and the individual clinical facility. Although documentation formats differ from facility to facility, all incorporate the professional and legal standards and criteria. The PTA should follow the policies and procedures of his or her clinical facility. Documenting according to professional standards and legal guidelines will produce a medical record that protects the patient and the PTA if the medical record is used in legal proceedings.

REFERENCES

1. Merriam-Webster Dictionary. Acessed March 15, 2006 at http://www.merriam-webster.com/dictionary.
2. American Physical Therapy Association. Direct access to physical therapy services. States that permit physical therapy treatment without referral. Accessed July 8, 2006 from http://www.apta.org/Advocacy/state/directaccess/State3.
3. Healthcare Finance Administration (HCFA), minimal data set (MDS), Regulations, HCFA/AMA documentation guidelines, home health regulations. Accessed March 29, 2007 from http://www.hcfa.gov.
4. Nagi, S. Z. (1969). *Disability and rehabilitation.* Columbus, OH: Ohio State University Press.
5. World Health Organization. (1980). *International classification of impairments, disabilities, and handicaps.* Geneva, Switzerland.
6. World Health Organization. (2001). *International classification of functioning, disability, and health.* Geneva, Switzerland.
7. National Center for Medical Rehabilitation Research. Accessed on March 29, 2007 from http://www.accessiblesociety.org/topics/demographics-identity/nidrr-lrp-defs.htm.
8. American Physical Therapy Association. (June 2003). Content, development and concepts. In *The guide to physical therapist practice* (pp. 19–25).
9. Medicare requirements. Accessed on March 29, 2007 from http://www.cms.hhs.gov.
10. American Physical Therapy Association. (June 2003). Standards of practice for physical therapy and the criteria. In *The guide to physical therapist practice* (pp. 685–688).
11. Comprehensive Accreditation Manual for Hospitals. (1996). Oakbrook Terrace, IL: Joint Commission on Accreditation of Healthcare Organizations (JCAHO).
12. Commission on Accreditation for Rehabilitation Facilities. Accessed on March 29, 2007 from http://www.carf.org.
13. American Physical Therapist Association. Accessed on March 29, 2007 from http://www.apta.org.

Review Exercises

1. Describe what is meant by the following rule: **"If it isn't written, it didn't happen."**

2. Describe the **changes** in referral for physical therapy that have occurred since the early 1960s.

3. Discuss how changes in referral for physical therapy **influenced** the evolution of the responsibilities of the PT and the PTA.

4. Define **documentation.** Give an example of how it is used in physical therapy.

5. Identify the **major factor** currently influencing the provision of health-care services and PT and PTA responsibilities.

6. Describe **three** purposes for the medical record.

7. Explain **why** the medical record can be audited.

8. **Who** determines standards or criteria for documentation?

9. Explain **why** the PTA should use the rule "follow the policies and procedures at the facility where you work."

10. From Figure 1–1, describe **why** this note is not appropriate as a record of today's patient care.

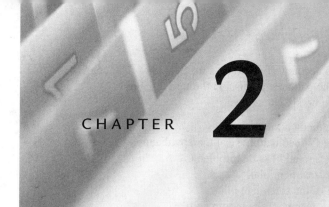

Documentation Content

LEARNING OBJECTIVES

After studying this chapter, the student will be able to:
- ☐ Identify the six categories of documentation content.
- ☐ Locate information in the medical record, based on the understanding of how medical record content is organized.
- ☐ Briefly describe the content to be documented in each category.
- ☐ Present documentation content in at least three different formats.
- ☐ Organize the information to be documented in a physical therapy note into a logical sequence.
- ☐ Differentiate between the medical diagnosis and the physical therapy diagnosis.
- ☐ Identify the five elements of physical therapy patient management.

INTRODUCTION   The medical record is the written account of a patient's medical care. The content describes the medical care provided from the patient's admission through discharge.

The content can be grouped into six categories:

1. The problem(s) requiring medical treatment
2. Data relevant to the patient's medical/physical therapy diagnosis
3. Treatment plan or action(s) to address the problem(s)
4. Goals or outcomes of the treatment plan
5. Record of administration of the treatment plan
6. Treatment effectiveness or results of the treatment plan

This information is found in written evaluations, progress notes, and specialized reports, such as those from the radiology department or clinical laboratory.

This chapter briefly describes each documentation category to provide an overview of the content of the medical record. In-depth explorations of these categories for physical therapy documentation are discussed in Chapters 3 through 6.

LOGICAL SEQUENCING OF CONTENT   The content provided in medical records can be organized using several different models. Most content organization models use a problem-solving approach to sequence the information. First, the data are gathered. Second, the data are interpreted and a judgment is made to identify the physical therapy diagnosis. Next, goals and outcomes are determined to direct the focus of physical therapy interventions. Finally, treatment plans designed to accomplish the goals and outcomes are outlined.

Five content models are used to teach PTAs how to organize and present the information describing the medical treatment and to determine what information is necessary. Medical facilities determine which model they will use on an individual basis:

1. SOAP (subjective, objective, assessment, and plan)
2. DEP (data, evaluation, performance)
3. PSPG (problem, status, plan, goals)
4. PSP (problem, status, plan)
5. Paragraph or narrative

Table 2–1 compares the organization models, their similarities and their methods of incorporating documentation content. Examples of the PSP, PSPG, and paragraph models are given in Figures 2–1, 2–2, and 2–3.

However, in any model used, it is the PT's responsibility to evaluate the patient and set the plan of care, and it is the PTA's responsibility to treat the patient within that plan of care. The PTA never sets the long-term goals but may have input into those goals through communications with the supervising PT.

Guidelines for Adapting to the Organization Models   The PTA can easily adapt to any organization model for the progress note by using the following problem-solving approach to sequence the information:

1. Introduce the progress note with a list or statement that tells the reader the physical therapy diagnoses for which the note is written.

Table 2–1 Comparing Organization Models				
Documentation Content	**SOAP**	**DEP**	**PSPG**	**PSP**
Problem	Pr	D	P	P
Subjective data	S	D	S	P
Objective data	O	D	S	S
Treatment effectiveness	A	E	S	S
Goals/outcomes	A	P	G	S
Plan	P	E	P	P

A = Assessment; D = Data; E = Evaluation; G = Goals; O = Objective data; P = Plan in SOAP and performance in DEP.
Pr = Problem; S = Subjective data in SOAP and Status in PSPG.

ABC Physical Therapy Clinic, Anytown, USA

June 1, 2006

P: 47 YOM, college math professor, Dx: chronic LBP syndrome; mild Ⓛ spine DJD; probable lumbar extension dysfunction; r/o HNP.

S: Pt. states, "I feel 50% better. The pain in my Ⓡ leg is gone now. I can sit for over an hour w/o any pain." Pt. attended back school on May 15, 2006. Exam: GMT/AROM WNL, ⒷLE, FAROM, Ⓛspine, w/o any c/o Sx. Neg. spasm, TTP, deformity. Neg. SLR to 85° Ⓑ, neg. Fabere. Gait, posture, SLR WNL. Performs extension exercises w/o difficulty or Sx.

P: Cont w/MH PRN, tid extension exercises, 10–15 reps. F/U w/ Dr. Brown scheduled for tomorrow. PT F/U 2–3 weeks or PRN. Pt. understands home program; pt. questions about exercise techniques answered.

Ron Therapist, PT

Figure 2–1 A note written in PSP organization. (Adapted from Scott, R. W. (1994). *Legal aspects of documenting patient care* (p. 79). Aspen, Gaithersburg, MD, with permission.)

2. Place the subjective and objective data first. Compare it with or relate it to the data in the initial or interim examination report.
3. Discuss the meaning of the data as it relates to treatment effectiveness and progress toward accomplishing the goals and functional outcomes listed in the initial or interim evaluation report.
4. Discuss the plan for future treatment sessions and involvement of the PT.

Several content organizations are illustrated for progress notes in Figures 2–1, 2–2, and 2–3. See Figure 1–2 in Chapter 1 for an example of a SOAP note.

FORMATS FOR THE PRESENTATION OF CONTENT

Information can be recorded using a variety of formats. Evaluations and progress notes may be either handwritten or dictated and typed. The progress notes may be narrative (i.e., written in paragraph form) or written in an outline format, such as the SOAP note. How the information in the medical record is organized depends on the preference of the medical facility. Each facility decides the format to use for recording data. The PTA must be familiar with the facility's charting procedures and must always follow the facility's policies, procedures, and format.

Computerized Documentation

Currently available computer software programs are designed for writing evaluations and progress notes. Many facilities have one or more computers in the department for the staff to use when documenting. A few facilities have a computer terminal in every hospital room or

---

Therapy Clinic, USA

June 1, 2006

P: 47 YOM, college math professor, Dx: chronic LBP syndrome; mild Ⓛ spine DJD; probable Lumbar extension dysfunction; r/o HNP.

S: Pt. was discharged as inpatient on May 5, 2006, and placed on OP home PT program of MH PRN and active extension exercises, tid X 10-15 reps. Today pt. states "I feel 50% better. The pain in my Ⓡ leg is gone now.
I can sit for over an hour w/o any pain." Pt. attended back school on May 15, 2006. Exam: GMT/AROM WNL, BLE, FAROM, Ⓛ spine, w/o any c/o Sx. Neg. spasm, TTP deformity. Neg. SLR to 85° Ⓑ, neg. Fabere. Gait, posture, SLT WNL. Performs extension exercises w/o difficulty or Sx.

P: Cont. w/MH PRN, tid extension exercise, 10-15 reps F/U w/ Dr. Brown scheduled for tomorrow. PT F/U 2-3 weeks or PRN. Pt. understands home program; pt. questions about exercise techniques answered.

G: Decrease residual Sx 50% X 2-3 wks; I pain-free ADL; prevent recurrence through good body mechanics.

Ron Therapist, PT

Figure 2–2 A note written in PSPG organization. This is a physical therapist's 4–week outpatient reevaluation form. (Adapted from Scott, R. W. (1994). *Legal aspects of documenting patient care* (p. 79). Aspen, Gaithersburg, MD, with permission.)

> **6-27-06: Dx: Status post pinned fractured R femur, dependent ambulation because of NWB on R leg.**
>
> Patient states he feels dizzy when he sits up but is eager to start walking on crutches and go home. Pt. c/o dizziness first time standing during treatment. Blood pressure before treatment 120/70 mmHg, first time up in // bars 108/65 mmHg, second standing trial 118/70 mmHg, after treatment 128/72 mmHg. Pt. responded to gait training with axillary crutches/minimal assist for sense of security and verbal cues for posture and heel contact/NWB on (R)/swing through gait 100 ft 2 X in hall, bed↔bathroom, and on carpet. Able to (I)sit↔stand with crutches from bed/lounge chair/toilet. Pt.'s progress toward functional outcome of community ambulation with crutches 50%. Blood pressure adjusting to upright position. Will teach stairs, ambulation on grass and car transfers tomorrow AM. Will notify PT discharge evaluation scheduled for tomorrow PM.
>
> Connie Competent,
> PTA Lic. #7890

Figure 2—3   Note combining all parts of a note given in a paragraph or narrative form.

in every treatment area of a physical therapy department. This allows the therapist to enter information in the patient's chart immediately after treatment. Physical therapy documentation software is advertised in publications such as *Physical Therapy* and *PT Magazine.* There are several examples available on the web, such as www.rehabdocumentation.com[1], www.theraclin.com[2], www.clinicient.com[3], and www.TheraSource.com.[4].

A word of warning is necessary about computerized documentation. This chapter discusses how the content of the progress note must be individualized to each patient, to clearly demonstrate how each patient is responding to the physical therapy treatment plan. Computerized documentation programs typically have preprogrammed statements or phrases that can be selected and combined to quickly compose the content of the progress note. The PTA must be careful that the selection of these phrases will clearly distinguish this patient from other patients and that the content will clearly describe the necessity for providing skilled physical therapy services. The software should allow the writer to type in his or her own words and phrases to individualize the note.

Flow Charts and Checklists

Much of the data, such as the patient's vital signs and functional status and the physical therapy interventions provided, can be recorded on flow charts, fill-in-the-blank forms, and checklists. By using these formats, the medical professional can easily visually scan the form to gather the information and quickly record the information in the chart. Hospitals, long-term-care facilities, and rehabilitation centers are facilities where the PTA will find narrative or outlined (commonly SOAP) notes, checklists, and flow charts. Figure 2–4 is an example of a flow chart for recording physical therapy treatments. Figure 2–5 illustrates two progress note forms combining a checklist or a flow chart with brief statements or a narration. A fill-in-the-blank form is depicted in Figure 2–6.

Letter Format

Physical therapists in private practice may communicate information about a patient to other medical professionals by letter. The data is recorded in the office by using any of the models already mentioned, but it is periodically summarized in letter format (Fig. 2–7). This type of format is commonly used when the patient's progress is being reported to a physician.

Individual Educational Program

In the public schools, physical therapy, occupational therapy, speech therapy, and psychological services provided to a student are planned and recorded in a format called an individual educational program (IEP). This format is in accordance with several laws passed by Congress relating to the provision of services to facilitate the education of students with disabilities. Professionals representing these services (e.g., teacher, OT, PT, school psychologist, speech pathologist) are included on the IEP team. The team records educational goals and objectives to be accomplished during the school year and holds meetings periodically to review the goals and objectives. It also meets with parents a minimum of every 6 months to make any needed changes. Box 2–1 lists the components of an IEP. These components are essentially the same as those of a physical therapy evaluation and progress note. Figure 2–8 is an example of the PT's contribution to the annual long-term goals and instructional objectives in an IEP written for a student. The PTA does not write the physical therapy goals and

DATE:

Orientation/Mood					
UE Strength/EX - bicep/tricep					
- W/C push up/rowing					
- shld flex/abd/horz abd/add					
TRANSPORT:					
- Transport to dept W/C/cart/amb					
Abductor pillow/knee immobilizer/prothesis/tilt tbl.					
- standing table					
GAIT: DEVICE:					
//bars; walker; crutches; cane; Qcane; none					
wt. bearing; NWB; TTWB; PWB; FWB; WBAT					
pattern: 2pt./3pt./4pt.					
distance/endurance					
Balance - sit/stand/walk					
Balance Act: lat/post/braid/line/sit/ball					
Stairs: rail/without rail/gait sequence					
TF's bed mobility					
toilet/raised seat/reg/commode bedside					
slidingboard transfer					
shower seat/car transfer					
supine → sit; sit → supine/sit to stand					
EX isometric quad, glut, HS, abd/ball squeeze					
ankle pump/circle/TB DF/PF/Ev/Inv					
hip flexion supine/sit/stand					
SLR flexion supine/stand					
SLR extension prone/stand/side lie					
SLR abduction supine/side lie/stand					
TKE supine/sit/SAQ/LAQ					
Bridging 1 leg/both					
knee AAROM sit/prone/supine					
KA PROM hip/knee/UE/ankle					
AAROM hip/knee/UE/ankle					
Stretching LE/UE					
Positional ROM/prone/long sit					
CPM					
Modalities H.P./ice/US/whirlpool					
Neuromusc. Re-Educ. Biofeed/CVA rehab					
HHA/Family instruction in:					
TF's-bed/toilet/shower/chair					
positioning/EX program					
walking program					
Written home program provided					
CHARGE - abbreviation for treatment					
THERAPIST					

SPC 337022   **REHABILITATION PHYSICAL THERAPY**

Restraints: NA/pelvic/vest

DNR Y/N

Precautions: _____

Figure 2—4   Flow chart form for recording physical therapy treatment.

objectives for the IEP but plays an important role by providing input for their planning. The PTA working in the school environment will document the progress being made toward accomplishing the physical therapy goals[5].

CARDEX   Within the physical therapy department, the patient's treatment goals and current intervention plan may be recorded in a cardex format. This 4×6-in. card is kept in a folder designed to hold many cards for quick access. The information is written in pencil so it can be updated easily. For example, in the morning the card may read that the patient ambulates from his bedroom to the nursing station and ambulates on the carpet in the lounge area. However, during the treatment session later in the afternoon, the patient ambulated past the station and to the stairs. The patient also managed three stairs for the first time. Now the information needs to be erased, and the new ambulation distance and the stair climbing must be described. When the PTA is treating a patient, he or she refers to the cardex information. Updating the information on a regular basis is essential to ensuring that the patient is progressing toward accomplishing the treatment goals. This cardex is to be used within the PT department; it is not a part of the patient's medical record. An intervention plan outlined on a cardex is depicted in Figure 2–9.

HOME CARE/HOSPICE SERVICES

Patient's Name:	Last		First		Age	Date	Time	Visit Frequency	Date Next Visit
Mood		Orientation		Cooperation		Communication	Pain		Rx Tolerance

		TREATMENTS			COMMENTS				
	Modalities	**WB Status**	**Ambulation**	**Exercise:**					
	Bed mobility	Non wt. bearing	Distance						
	Elec. stim.	Partial	Assist.						
	Ex. active	Toe touch	Balance						
	Ex ROM	Full	Coord.						
	Ex back	Non amb.	Pattern						
	Ex breathing		Stairs						
	Ex coord.								
	Ex isometric	**Equipment**	**Transfers**	**Problems/Progess:**					
	Ex man. resist	Walker	Bed						
	Ex mm re-ed.	Crutches	Toilet						
	Ex PRE	Cane	Tub						
	Ex gait tmg.		Chair						
	Massage		Car						
	Packs	**ROM**							
	Stump wrap								
	Transfers		Other						
	Tx								
	Ultrasound								
	Evaluation								
	MD contact								
	Instruction		**Follow-through/Response:**						
	Patient								
	Support Person								
	HHA								

THERAPIST SIGNATURE

Figure 2—5A   Physical therapy progress note forms that combine presentation styles. This form combines a checklist with brief statements.

Physical Therapy Daily Progress Notes						
MODALITIES:	DATE/Initials	DATE/Initials	DATE/Initials	DATE/Initials	DATE/Initials	DATE/Initials
Hot Pack/Cold Packs						
Massage/Ice Massage						
Electrical Stimulation						
Traction						
Ultrasound						
Kinetic Activity						
Therapeutic Exercise						
Neuromuscular Re-ed						
Functional Activities						
Training in ADL's						
Serial Casting						
Gait Training						
Orthotics/Prosthetics Train.						
Wound Care						
Whirlpool Therapy						
Conference						
Consultation						
Other						

Date	Comments:

Assessment:

Goals:

Plan:

_____		_____
(Name)	Date	

_____		
(Name)	Date	

_____		
(Name)	Date	

Treatment Diagnosis:

Figure 2—5B Physical therapy progress note forms that combine presentation styles. This form combines a flow chart with narration.

Level of Independence	Without Help	Uses Device	Help of Another	Device and Help	Dependent/ Does Not Do	Not Determined
Feeding						
Hygiene/Grooming						
Transfers						
Homemaking						
Bath/Shower						
Dressing						
Bed Mobility						
Home Mgt.						

Physical Environment: _____

_____

Psychosocial: _____

Safety Measures: _____

_____

Equipment in Home: _____

Emergency No: _____ *Nutritional Req: _____ Allergies: _____

Unusual Home/Social Environment: _____

*Known Medical Reason Pt. leaves home: _____

Other Services Involved: _____ Prognosis: _____

Vulnerable Adult Assessment: _____ Low Risk _____ High Risk _____

Caregiver Status: _____

Pulse: _____   BP: _____

Current Medications: _____   _____

_____   _____

_____   _____

Patient's Prior Status: _____

_____

Scheduled MD Follow-up Appt(s): _____

_____

Name: _____

Rx#: _____

Figure 2—6   Form with a fill-in-the blank format.

July 21, 2006
RE: Mr. Tom Jones
Dx: Femur Fx

Update on Progress:

Mr. Jones is making good progress recovering from the fracture of the (L) femur. Patient is now able to ambulate 100 feet with a quad cane and SBA, 4x/day. Pt. has full AROM in (L) LE and strength is 4/5 in all muscles. Recommend continued therapy 2x/week with continuation of daily home program.

Figure 2—7   Example of a letter format.

Learner's Name:	
Annual Goals, Short-term Instructional Objectives	
Thoroughly state the goal. List objectives for the goal, including attainment criteria for each objective.	Goal #_____ of _____ Goals

Goal:

The student will independently move about the school building and within the classroom using a wheelchair to participate in all daily school activities, and the student will independently transfer from wheelchair to desk seat, to floor for participation and position change in 6 months.

Short-term Instructional Objectives

1. The student will independently open doors to the gymnasium and maneuver the wheelchair through the entrance to the gym 1/3 trials in 3 months.
2. The student will independently transfer from wheelchair to floor and back into the chair 1/3 trials in 3 months.
3. The student will safely and independently maneuver the wheelchair around the tables in the cafeteria 1/3 trials in 3 months.

IEP Periodic Review

Date Reviewed: _____
Progress made toward this goal and objective

The learner's IEP

☐ Meets learner's current needs and will be continued without changes.

☐ Does not meet learner's current needs and the modifications (not significant) listed below will be made without an IEP meeting unless you contact us.

☐ Does not meet learner's current needs and the significant changes listed below require a revised IEP. We will be in contact soon to schedule a meeting.

Note to Parent(s): You are entitled to request a meeting to discuss the results of this review.

Figure 2—8   An example of the PT's contribution to the goals and instructional objectives on an individual education program (IEP) written for a child in school.

Box 2-1   Components of an IEP

1. A statement of the student's current levels of educational performance.
2. A statement of annual goals, including short-term instructional objectives.
3. A statement of the specific special education and related services to be provided to the student and the extent to which the child will be able to participate in regular education programs.
4. The projected dates for initiation of services and the anticipated duration of the services.
5. Appropriate objective criteria and evaluation procedures and schedules for determining on at least an annual basis, whether the short-term instructional objectives are being achieved (34CFR 300.334).

From American Physical Therapy Association and the Section on Pediatrics: Individualized educational program and individualized family service plan. In Martin, KD (ed): Physical Therapy Practice in Educational Environments; Policies and Guidelines, APTA. Alexandria, VA. 1990,p.6.I.

DX: R CVA with hemiplegia

INITIAL DATE: 2-24-06

PRECAUTIONS: Broca's Aphasia, feeding tube

UPDATE: 3-20-06

Exercise	Set	Rep	Equipment	Assist	Goals
PROM/AAROM Ⓛ UE & LE, prone	1	10		muscle belly	1. Ⓘ bed mobility
Knee flexion	1	10	1# cuff weight	tapping	2. Ⓘ unsupported sit
TKE long sit	1	10	2# cuff weight	verbal cues	3. Ⓘ w/c mobility
	1	as many as he can; goal of 10 reps			4. Standing pivot transfer with min assist of 1
	2	10	2# cuff weight	verbal cues	
	2	10	2# cuff weight		**TDD:**
Standing 10 min; work on eye tracking and lip closure	2	10	1# cuff weight	Standing table	**TDP:**

Patient's Name	Age	Sex	MD	PT	RM#	Unit
Henry I.	**71**	**M**	**Smith**	**Jones**	**E123**	**12**

Transfers	Method	Assist	Other
bed↔w/c, w/c↔mat, w/c↔toilet w/c↔straight chair	Stand pivot to Ⓡ side	Max. x 1	Practice squat pivot transfer w/c↔mat moving towards Ⓛ.

Pregait/Gait

Stand in//bars-max assist x 1 – midline with mirror and wt. shifting to Ⓛ. Watch Ⓛ knee – no hyperextension.

Sitting balance in w/c with arms removed and in armless straight chair. Min assist x 2. Work on head movement, eye tracking, wt. shifting, and trunk rot.

W/c mobility – room to bathroom, room to dining room, to PT, OT and Speech departments. Check seating/cushion, Ⓛ scapula protracted, and arm on tray.

Figure 2–9   A treatment plan outlined on a cardex, commonly used in physical therapy departments to keep treatment procedures current.

Standardized Medicare Forms

Standardized Medicare forms are used to chart the medical care given to patients covered by Medicare. The Health Care Financing Administration specifies the format and time lines for recording and submitting data. The Medicare Plan of Treatment for Outpatient Rehabilitation and the Updated Plan of Progress for Rehabilitation forms (Forms CMS-700 and -701, see Figs. 2–10, 2–11) are intended to be evaluation forms. These forms should **not** be completed by a PTA.[6]

The approval for physical therapy services is periodically renewed or recertified (at present, every 30 days). When the PT recommends that therapy be continued for the patient to meet the goals, this form becomes an interim evaluation. If the patient has reached maximum benefit or has met the goals, this form serves as a discharge evaluation. The PTA can provide the PT with information about the status of the patient, but the PT completes the form.

Narrative

A narrative reporting format describes the treatment session with the patient in a more "descriptive" manner and does not provide the type of structure you might find in other formats. This type of reporting is used to describe short treatment sessions with a patient or any type of interaction with other health-care personnel responsible for the patient's care. This type of note can review a simple treatment session, document a brief discussion with another health-care worker regarding the patient's treatment session or progress, or provide a simple discussion of the patient's progress. Again, this type of note may be easier to construct, but because it is less structured, important information may be omitted.

Templates

Templates are forms developed by a medical facility to shorten the patient documentation time and to ensure a more orderly and complete reporting process by all employees. These forms can be developed in a computer module or on paper. Various companies now provide these types of documentation materials, and many of the larger facilities tend to use them. When using this type of a format, several problems that develop relate to the inability of the therapist to provide any detailed narrative that may ensure quality patient care. This format also makes it difficult for students and new therapists to develop the skills necessary for quality reporting of patient care.

ORGANIZATION OF THE MEDICAL RECORD

Until the 1970s, hospitals typically used the source-oriented method for organizing the medical record. In the 1970s, the problem-oriented method was introduced, offering another way to organize information. The PTA who has the opportunity to gain work experience in several different clinical facilities may see both types of records. More commonly, however, facilities use variations and combinations of source-oriented and problem-oriented organizations. Today, the PTA may be recording in medical records organized according to the functional abilities of the patient.

Source-Oriented Medical Record

The source-oriented medical record (SOMR) is organized according to the medical services offered by the clinical facility. A section in the chart is labeled with a tab marker or color-coded for each discipline. For example, the SOMR might be organized with the physician's section first, followed by sections for nursing, physical therapy, occupational therapy, and then test results. Caregivers in each discipline document their content (e.g., data, problems, treatment plans, goals, progress notes, and treatment effectiveness) in the section designated for their discipline. The sections must be clearly marked for easy identification so the reader can locate the information. Source-oriented organization is criticized because the time required to read through each section for information makes the record difficult to audit for reimbursement and quality control.

Each professional on the medical team should be responsible for reading the chart frequently, communicating with other medical professionals, and staying informed about the patient's latest treatments and condition. Professionals in one discipline might identify a patient's problem and begin treatment, whereas professionals in the rest of the disciplines may not be aware that the problem exists. For example, a nurse discovers high blood pressure and obtains medication orders from the physician. The nurse records this information in the section for nursing notes. The patient experiences side effects from this new medication that

DEPARTMENT OF HEALTH AND HUMAN SERVICES
CENTERS FOR MEDICARE & MEDICAID SERVICES

PLAN OF TREATMENT FOR OUTPATIENT REHABILITATION
(COMPLETE FOR INITIAL CLAIMS ONLY)

1. PATIENT'S LAST NAME	FIRST NAME	M.I.	2. PROVIDER NO.	3. HICN

4. PROVIDER NAME	5. MEDICAL RECORD NO. *(Optional)*	6. ONSET DATE	7. SOC. DATE

8. TYPE	9. PRIMARY DIAGNOSIS *(Pertinent Medical D.X.)*	10.TREATMENT DIAGNOSIS	11. VISITS FROM SOC.
☐ PT ☐ OT ☐ SLP ☐ CR ☐ RT ☐ PS ☐ SN ☐ SW			

12. PLAN OF TREATMENT FUNCTIONAL GOALS

GOALS *(Short Term)*

OUTCOME *(Long Term)*

PLAN

13. SIGNATURE *(professional establishing POC including prof. designation)*	14. FREQ/DURATION *(e.g., 3/Wk. x 4 Wk.)*

I CERTIFY THE NEED FOR THESE SERVICES FURNISHED UNDER THIS PLAN OF TREATMENT AND WHILE UNDER MY CARE   ☐ N/A

15. PHYSICIAN SIGNATURE	16. DATE

17. CERTIFICATION
FROM   THROUGH   N/A

18. ON FILE *(Print/type physician's name)*
☐

20. INITIAL ASSESSMENT *(History, medical complications, level of function at start of care. Reason for referral.)*

19. PRIOR HOSPITALIZATION
FROM   TO   N/A

21. FUNCTIONAL LEVEL *(End of billing period)* PROGRESS REPORT   ☐ CONTINUE SERVICES **OR**   ☐ DC SERVICES

22. SERVICE DATES
FROM   THROUGH

Form CMS-700-(11-91)

Figure 2—10   Medicare Plan of Treatment for Outpatient Rehabilitation Form CMS-700.

DEPARTMENT OF HEALTH AND HUMAN SERVICES
CENTERS FOR MEDICARE & MEDICAID SERVICES

UPDATED PLAN OF PROGRESS FOR OUTPATIENT REHABILITATION
(Complete for Interim to Discharge Claims. Photocopy of CMS-700 or 701 is required.)

1. PATIENT'S LAST NAME	FIRST NAME	M.I.	2. PROVIDER NO.	3. HICN

4. PROVIDER NAME	5. MEDICAL RECORD NO. *(Optional)*	6. ONSET DATE	7. SOC. DATE

8. TYPE ☐ PT ☐ OT ☐ SLP ☐ CR ☐ RT ☐ PS ☐ SN ☐ SW	9. PRIMARY DIAGNOSIS *(Pertinent Medical D.X.)*	10. TREATMENT DIAGNOSIS	11. VISITS FROM SOC.
	12. FREQ/DURATION *(e.g., 3/Wk. x 4 Wk.)*		

13. CURRENT PLAN UPDATE, FUNCTIONAL GOALS *(Specify changes to goals and plan.)*

GOALS *(Short Term)*   PLAN

OUTCOME *(Long Term)*

I HAVE REVIEWED THIS PLAN OF TREATMENT AND RECERTIFY A CONTINUING NEED FOR SERVICES. ☐ N/A ☐ DC

14. RECERTIFICATION
FROM   THROUGH   N/A

15. PHYSICIAN'S SIGNATURE	16. DATE	17. ON FILE *(Print/type physician's name)* ☐

18. REASON(S) FOR CONTINUING TREATMENT THIS BILLING PERIOD *(Clarify goals and necessity for continued skilled care.)*

19. SIGNATURE *(or name of professional, including prof. designation)*	20. DATE	21. ☐ CONTINUE SERVICES **OR** ☐ DC SERVICES

22. FUNCTIONAL LEVEL *(At end of billing period — Relate your documentation to functional outcomes and list problems still present.)*

22. SERVICE DATES
FROM   THROUGH

Form CMS-701(11-91)

Figure 2—11   Medicare Recertification Form CMS-701.

affect his or her ability to fully understand the PTA's exercise instructions. If the PTA has not taken the time to read the nursing section of the patient's chart and is unaware of this additional medication, the PTA may incorrectly assume and document in the physical therapy's section that the patient is being uncooperative today. To ensure communication and coordination among the health-care providers, regular meetings are necessary so medical personnel can gather to discuss the patient's problems and progress. A written record of these meetings should be placed in the patient's chart.

Problem-Oriented Medical Record

In the 1970s, Dr. Lawrence Weed introduced the problem-oriented medical record (POMR) as an attempt to eliminate the disadvantages associated with SOMR. Content in this type of medical record is organized around identification and treatment of the patient's problems. The components or sections of the POMR are organized in the following sequence, thus ordering information about the patient's medical care from admission to discharge:

1. Database
2. Problem list
3. Treatment plans
4. Progress notes
5. Discharge notes

Each section contains the appropriate information from each discipline. For example, the data gathered by the physician, PT, and OT are recorded in the database section. For each of these disciplines, the problems identified are listed in the problem list section, the treatment plans in the treatment plan section, and the progress notes in the progress note section. Each caregiver may record on the same page within each section. Alternatively, subsections may be designated for each discipline within the main sections of the POMR.

Communication among disciplines is enhanced because the problems identified and treated by each discipline are all in one place. The organization also allows specific information, such as the treatment results, to be found easily should the record be audited.

Functional Outcome Report

Swanson[7] proposed the use of the functional outcome report (FOR), a structured approach for reporting functional assessment and outcomes (Box 2–2). The sequence of the information in the FOR is as follows:

1. Reason for referral
2. Functional limitations
3. Physical therapy assessment
4. Therapy problems
5. Functional outcome goals
6. Treatment plan and rationale

The reason for referral section includes the medical diagnosis, past medical history, and subjective data. The functional limitations and physical therapy assessment sections contain the objective data. The physical problems are identified based on the data. The functional goals are listed, and the report concludes with the treatment plan and how it relates to accomplishing the functional goals.

SOAP Notes

SOAP notes are perhaps the most widely used type of documentation, and the documentation most commonly used in the 1970s and 1980s before the widespread use of computers. This type of documentation provides the new therapist and the student with an outline type of format to document what happens during the patient treatment session. It also provides the individual therapist with a means of chronicling what has happened with the patient during each treatment session, the patient's progress, and recommendations for continuing care. This type of format provides the beginning therapist with an organized method to outline what they hear from the patient, to provide measurable goals, to analyze the treatment session, and to plan for continued treatment and referral to other health-care providers. See Box 2–3 for an exam-

---

Box 2-2   Example of an Initial Functional Outcome Report

Reason for Referral

Patient post meniscectomy of left knee reports pain, stiffness, and difficulty with walking and other upright mobility activities.

Functional Limitations

Activity	Current Status
Sit-to-stand transfer	Independent
Standing balance	Performs independently, with cane
Flat terrain ambulation (speed)	Performs with cane for more than 18 sec for 20 ft
Flat terrain ambulation (endurance)	Tolerates less than 5 min
Ambulation on uneven terrain	Unable
Stair climbing	Ascends two steps, descends two steps with railing and minimum assistance

PT Assessment

Medical diagnosis status post meniscectomy is further defined to include residual left knee joint inflammation.

Positive test findings: Positive fluctuation test; limited strength; quadriceps 3/5 and hamstring 4/5, indicative of synovial effusion.

Therapy Problems

1. Pain on compression maneuvers of the left knee: sitting sit to stance, periodically during gait cycle, during all phases of stair climbing.
2. Difficulty in coordinating gait cycle with use of cane to reduce stress to left knee.

Functional Outcome Goals

Activity	Performance	Due Date
Flat terrain ambulation (speed)	Independent without device; 20 ft in 9 sec	Within 14 days
Flat terrain ambulation (endurance)	Tolerates unassisted walking for 30 min	Within 21 days
Uneven terrain ambulation	Tolerates for a minimum of 15 min	Within 14 days
Stair climbing	Ascends and descends 15 steps	Within 21 days

Treatment Plan with Rationale

Application of anti-inflammatory modalities with instruction for follow-up home program to minimize post-activity edema.

Lower extremity strength training with instruction in progressive home exercise program.

Patient instructed in activity limits and restrictions during the course of care.

From Swanson, G: Functional Outcome Report: The next generation in physical therapy reporting. In Steward, D, and Abein, 5 (eds). Documenting Functional Outcomes in Physical Therapy, Mosby Yearbook, St. Louis, MO, 1993.

---

ple of each section of the SOAP note. It is one of the simplest documentation methods used and will be discussed, in detail, in Chapters 3 through 6.

ORGANIZATION OF THE DOCUMENTATION CONTENT

Clinical facilities often differ in the way their documentation is organized and sequenced within the evaluation reports and progress notes. A study of some examples of content organization models reveals a common logic to the sequencing of the information.

> **Box 2–3   SOAP Note Format**
>
> **S:** This section includes subjective types of information reported by the patient, family, caretakers, or other health-care providers that are related to the patient's treatment and response to the treatment.
>
> **O:** This section includes all the objective types of information, including specific measurements, range of motion, strength ratings, functional levels, tone, therapeutic exercises, number of repetitions and sets of exercises, and any other measurable treatment protocols.
>
> **A:** This section contains assessment information related to the patient's response to the treatment session, a summary of how the session was conducted and completed, and the introduction of a home program with a review and changes in patient status.
>
> **P:** This section contains the continued plan for treatment, communication with the supervising PT, recommendations for the supervisory visit, and recommendations for any necessary referrals or plans for discharge to another facility or to the patient's home.

Problem, Status, Plan, (PSP); Problem, Status, Plan, Goals (PSPG); and Data, Evaluation, Performance Goals (DEP) Models

A model more typically used for the progress note or interim evaluation report is the PSP (mnemonic for Problem, Status, Plan), a variation of the SOAP note. The patient's physical therapy problem/diagnosis and medical diagnosis are stated under the first P section. Subjective and objective data about the patient's condition at the time of the interim evaluation are documented under the S section. The second P section contains the modified treatment plan indicated by the clinical findings. The PSPG model adds a G section for functional goals. Review Figures 2–1 and 2–2 for examples of notes in PSP and PSPG models.[8]

Another model for organizing and documenting information is DEP (mnemonic for data, evaluation, performance goals), a model for performance-based documentation designed by El-Din and Smith.[9] The subjective and objective data (D) are combined into one section. In the evaluation section (E), data is interpreted and physical therapy diagnoses are identified; the treatment plan also is included in this section. The performance goals (P) section contains the functional goals for treatment and the expected time frame for meeting these goals.

THE PROBLEM REQUIRING MEDICAL TREATMENT

The medical team identifies the patient's medical problems on the basis of the data collected by the various disciplines. The physician determines the medical diagnosis (Dx), and other professionals identify problems that are treatable within their respective disciplines. The diagnosis is documented by the physician in the medical chart, usually near the beginning of the chart in a section specified for the physician's report. The identification of the physical therapy problem, called the physical therapy diagnosis (PT Dx), is usually documented in the physical therapy initial evaluation, located in either the physical therapy section or the evaluation section of the chart. The diagnosis documented by the physician may be different than the one used in the physical therapy diagnosis, depending on the patient's medical history. Other problems are discussed in other health-care providers' evaluations. In the example of the student in the motorcycle accident, (see Table 2–2) possible problems identified by the physicians, nurses, and social worker may include the following:

1. Compound fracture of the shaft of the right femur
2. Lacerations into the quadriceps muscles
3. Infected open wound
4. Edema of the right foot
5. Questionable chemical dependency
6. Fever
7. Elevated blood pressure

DEFINITION OF TERMS

Some terms need to be defined before comparing the medical diagnoses with the physical therapy diagnosis. The preferred practice patterns of physical therapy outlined by the APTA

Table 2-2	Examples of Data Gathered by Various Services for a Patient in a Motorcycle Accident	

Discipline/Service	Data
Admitting clerk	Past admission to the hospital
	Insurance information
	Nearest relative
	General information about the accident
Physician	Past medical history
	Detailed information about the accident
	Physical examination
	Orthopedic examination results from orthopedic surgeon
	Diagnostic and laboratory test results, such as x-rays
Nurse	Vital signs
	Bowel and bladder function
	Skin condition
	General nutritional status
	General ability for self-care, communication, and decision-making
Physical therapist	Flexibility or joint range of motion
	Muscle strength
	Sensation
	Posture
	Ability to move about in environment
	Functional level (pre and post)
Occupational therapist	Specific ability for self-care in activities of daily living
	Vocational abilities
	Homemaking abilities
	General vision, hearing, and communication abilities
Social worker	Home environment and lifestyle
	More specific financial concerns
	General emotional development
	Family support and family adjustment

in *The Guide to Physical Therapist Practice** are based on a process of disablement. This process describes a chain of events beginning with a pathology, which may lead to impairments, which may then lead to functional limitations, and which may result in a disability. *Impairment* is defined as "loss or abnormality of physiological, psychological, or anatomical structure or function." *Functional limitation* is "restriction of the ability to perform—at the level of the whole person—a physical action, activity, or task in an efficient, typically expected, or competent manner." *Disability* refers to "the inability to engage in age-specific, gender-specific, or sex-specific roles in a particular social context and physical environment." More broadly, disability can be defined as a general term that refers to any long- or short-term reduction of a person's activity as a result of an acute or chronic condition.[10]

This disablement framework is a variation of the framework describing the implication of pathology issued by the World Health Organization (WHO). The terminology in this model, the International Classification of Impairments, Disabilities, and Handicaps (ICIDH-2), is used in the international physical therapy community. The ICIDH-2 provides a framework and an international common language for the organization and compilation of disability data, the international comparison of these data, and forms the basis for assessment instruments. The ICIDH-2 term disability is equivalent to APTA's functional limitation, and the ICIDH-2 term handicap has the same meaning as APTA's disability. In 2001, WHO changed the terminology used in the ICIDH and a new version, ICIDH-2, was introduced (see Fig. 2–12). The new proposal is ICIDH-2.[11]

This new terminology is in line with the APTA's definitions of impairment, functional limitation, and disability. These three sections are further defined in a checklist provided with

---

International Classification of Functioning and Disability

" 'Functioning' and 'disability' are umbrella terms covering three dimensions: (1) body functions and structure; (2) activities at the individual level; and (3) participation in society."[12a]

Figure 2—12   International Classification of Functioning and Disability.

the new version of the ICIDH-2. To complete the *Checklist,* the clinician can use a series of structured interview questions, referred to as *General Questions for Participation and Activities,* to obtain relevant information from patients. This information is then used for "rating" or "qualifying" the patient's activity and participation and the environmental factors affecting the individual on the *Checklist.*

Through the use of this *Checklist,* a patient's disability or impairment in function can help determine the extent of the impairment, the nature of the change introduced into the patient's life because of this impairment, the performance qualifier (the extent of participation restriction), and the capacity qualifier (the extent of activity limitation).

The **Checklist** includes the following rankings:

1. *Mild impairment* means a problem that is present less than 25% of the time, with an intensity a person can tolerate, and that happened rarely over the last 30 days.
2. *Moderate impairment* means a problem that is present less than 50% of the time, with an intensity that is interfering in the person's day-to-day life, and that happened occasionally over the last 30 days.
3. *Severe impairment* means a problem that is present more than 50% of the time, with an intensity that is partially disrupting the person's day-to-day life, and that happened frequently over the last 30 days.
4. *Complete impairment* means a problem that is present more than 95% of the time, with an intensity that is totally disrupting the person's day-to-day life, and that happened every day over the last 30 days.
5. *Not specified* means there is insufficient information to specify the severity of the impairment.
6. *Not applicable* means it is inappropriate to apply a particular code (e.g., b650 Menstruation functions for women of premenarche or postmenopause age).

Included within the functional definitions should be some reference to "prior level of function (PLOF)" and "current level of function (CLOF)" to determine the difference between the patient's abilities preincident and postincident.[11]

MEDICAL DIAGNOSIS

The medical diagnosis is of a systemic disease or disorder that is determined by the physician's evaluation and diagnostic tests. "Diagnosis is the recognition of disease. It is the determination of the cause and nature of pathologic conditions."[12] The medical diagnosis is equivalent to the pathology in the APTA and the ICIDH-2 frameworks. In the example of the student in the motorcycle accident (see Table 2–2), the medical diagnosis was "a fractured femur and infected lacerations."

PHYSICAL THERAPY PROBLEM DIAGNOSIS

The physical therapy problem is not a medical diagnosis. According to Sahrmann,[13] the physical therapy problem is the identification of pathokinesiologic (i.e., study of movements related to a given disorder) problems associated with faulty biomechanical or neuromuscular action. In Sahrmann's definition, faulty biomechanical or neuromuscular action is termed *impairments,* and pathokinesiologic problems are called *functional limitations.*

In the APTA's model, the physical therapy diagnosis consists of the patient's impairments and functional limitations; whereas in the ICIDH-2 model, the physical therapy diagnosis consists of the patient's impairments and disabilities. In both models, the physical therapy treatment objectives are aimed at eliminating or minimizing the impairments and functional limitations or disabilities. The desired outcome of the physical therapy treatment is preventing or minimizing the severity of the disability or handicap.

Impairments. Impairments are abnormalities or dysfunctions of the bones, joints, ligaments, muscles, tendons, nerves, and skin, or problems with movement resulting from a pathology in the brain, spinal cord, pulmonary, or cardiovascular systems. A few common examples of dysfunctions treatable by physical therapy include muscle weakness; tendon inflammation; connective tissue tightness with limited range of motion (ROM) in the joints; muscle spasms; edema; and difficulties moving in bed, moving from sitting to standing, and walking. Impairments in the physical therapy diagnosis may be the same as in the medical diagnosis, such as "a rotated L5 vertebra" with muscle spasms and pain limiting a truck driver's sitting tolerance to 5 minutes. The physician, after determining that the L5 vertebra is rotated on the basis of x-rays and examination, may indicate this as the medical diagnosis. If the patient went to see the PT first, the PT, after performing the examination, may identify the rotated vertebra. This, plus the muscle spasms, is the musculoskeletal dysfunction part of the physical therapy diagnosis. A patient may have a medical diagnosis with a physical therapy diagnosis, such as rheumatoid arthritis with adhesive capsulitis of the anterior capsule limiting shoulder ROM interfering with a retiree's ability to put on shirt and sweater. In the latter case, rheumatoid arthritis is the medical diagnosis, and adhesive capsulitis limiting shoulder ROM is part of the physical therapy diagnosis.

Functional Limitations. The definition of the physical therapy diagnosis must include the patient's functional abilities or inabilities. The patient comes to physical therapy because of an inability to function adequately in his or her environment. In the previously cited examples, the patient with the fractured femur will not be able to ambulate bearing weight on the fractured leg, the truck driver with the rotated L5 vertebra cannot sit longer than 5 minutes, and the retiree with rheumatoid arthritis cannot put on his shirt and sweater. These functional problems become the basis for determining the outcomes toward which the physical therapy treatments are directed, and the rate of progress toward accomplishing the goals and outcomes determines the duration of the physical therapy services.[12]

Differentiation Between the Medical Diagnosis and Physical Therapy Diagnosis

The PTA should distinguish between the medical diagnosis and the physical therapy diagnosis when treating and documenting. Examples of medical diagnoses include the following:

1. Multiple sclerosis
2. Rheumatoid arthritis
3. Fractured right femur
4. Cerebral vascular accident secondary to thrombosis
5. Compression fracture of T12 vertebra with compression of spinal cord

Physical therapy diagnoses that may be associated with the medical diagnoses listed above are discussed in Box 2–4.

TREATMENT PLANS OR ACTIONS

The list of the patient's medical problems is used to plan the patient's medical treatment. Appropriate strategies for resolving or minimizing the problems are outlined by the various disciplines involved. These strategies are the treatment plans. In the case of the motorcycle accident patient (see Table 2–2), the physician would design a treatment plan for medication to stop the infection and then for surgery to pin and stabilize the fractured femur. Nursing may design a treatment plan for positioning the right foot to reduce the edema and for monitoring blood pressure. The social worker may design a treatment plan to help the patient address his questionable chemical dependency. Later, the PT may design a treatment plan to teach the patient to walk with crutches. In the previous example of the truck driver, the PT may design a treatment plan to include applying a physical agent to relax muscle spasms, performing mobilization techniques to derotate the L5 vertebra, and educating the driver about sitting support and posture. These treatment plans, described in the medical record, include the frequency and duration of the treatment procedures.

Informed Consent to the Treatment Plan

All aspects of the treatment plan, including the purposes, procedures, expected results, and any possible risks or side effects of treatment, must be explained to the patient and significant others. In some cases, the patient may participate in designing the plan. The patient or a representative for the patient should agree to the treatment plan and procedures. His or her

---

Box 2–4   Physical Therapy versus Medical Diagnosis

Physical Therapy Diagnosis
Ataxia of lower extremities with inability to ambulate independently.

Discussion
A patient with the medical diagnosis of multiple sclerosis may have the physical therapy diagnosis of ataxia (the impairment) and the functional problem of inability to ambulate (the functional limitation). In the past, the result of the treatment was documented by a description of the improvement in impairment (e.g., pt.'s coordination improved as pt. able to place Ⓡ heel on Ⓛ knee). Today, treatment effectiveness is documented by a description of a decrease in the functional limitation, such as improvement in the ability or quality of the patient's ambulation (e.g., pt. able to walk to mailbox without assistive device but needs standby assist because of occasional loss of balance).

Physical Therapy Diagnosis
ROM deficits in right shoulder limiting the ability to put on shirt and sweater.

Discussion
The patient with the medical diagnosis of rheumatoid arthritis may have the physical therapy diagnosis consisting of the impairment, ROM deficits, and the functional limitation (APTA) or disability (ICIDH-2) of difficulty in dressing. In the past, it was acceptable to document treatment effectiveness in degrees of increased ROM (e.g., shoulder flexion 0°–100°, an improvement of 20° since initial evaluation). Today, a description of the patient's ability to put on his or her shirt or sweater, along with the improvement in degrees of ROM, documents the treatment effectiveness (e.g., patient able to put on loose-fitting pullover sweater without assistance) and puts meaning to the ROM degrees.

---

decision to consent to the treatment (informed consent) is based on the information provided about the treatment. In many medical facilities, a formal informed consent form or document must be signed before treatment is initiated. When a patient is receiving physical therapy, the PT designs the treatment plan and reviews the plan with the patient. Thus, the appropriate person to obtain the informed consent signature is the PT, not the PTA. Once signed, this form is placed in the medical record.[8]

GOALS AND OUTCOMES

All health-care providers identify the goals or outcomes to be accomplished by their treatment plans. In the case of the student involved in the motorcycle accident (see Table 2–2), the physician's goals may be to treat the infection and stabilize the fractured femur so healing can occur. The nurse's goals may be to monitor the patient and prevent any other problems as a result of the patient's injury and temporary inactivity. The social worker's goal may be to help the patient find the most appropriate resources and help for his chemical dependency.

The functional outcomes toward which the PT's treatment plan is directed should include the patient's expectations (i.e., what is meaningful to the patient) for eliminating or minimizing the patient's functional limitations. The physical therapy goals are directed toward eliminating or minimizing the patient's impairments.

Therefore, the physical therapy goals and outcomes are planned with patient and PT collaboration. The goals for the truck driver are to decrease his pain and improve his trunk ROM, whereas his functional outcome is to be able to sit for at least 2 hours so he can return to work.

The student's functional outcome is to learn how to use crutches so he can return to college. The goals and outcomes give the PTA direction for planning the treatment sessions, progressing the treatment outlined in the PT's plan, and recommending the termination of treatment. The PT and the PTA need to stay focused on the purpose of the treatment plan, gearing everything done during a treatment session toward improving or resolving the functional problem that brought the client to physical therapy. Likewise, all documentation should be focused on the treatment appropriate for the goals and outcomes and on the progress toward accomplishing the functional outcomes.

RECORD OF ADMINISTRATION OF THE TREATMENT PLAN

The medical chart contains proof that the treatment plan is being carried out. Recording the administration of the treatment procedures can range from simply checking off items listed in a flow chart or checklist to writing a narration or report about the treatment in daily, weekly, or monthly progress notes.

Progress Note

The progress note is a recording of the treatment provided for each problem, the patient's reaction to the treatment procedures and progress toward goals and outcomes, and any changes in the patient's condition. Although both the PT and the PTA write the progress notes, this text is directed toward the skills needed by the PTA to write quality notes.

TREATMENT EFFECTIVENESS

The treatment effectiveness content contains an interpretation of the patient's response to the treatment. It is the *most* important content in the medical record and is considered the "bottom line" of the health-care business. Here, the therapist documents whether or not goals were met, thus documenting the effectiveness of the treatment plan. This information tells the reader about the quality of the medical care provided. The researcher uses this content to measure outcomes and determine the efficacy of treatment procedures. The third-party payer reads this information to determine whether the medical care met the requirements for reimbursement.

THE EXAMINATION AND EVALUATION BY PHYSICAL THERAPY

According to *The Guide to Physical Therapist Practice,* "the physical therapist integrates five elements of patient/client management—examination, evaluation, diagnosis, prognosis, and intervention—in a manner designed to maximize outcomes (Figure 2–13)."[10]

Five Elements of Physical Therapy Patient Management

Examination is the process for gathering subjective and objective data about the patient. *Evaluation* is the clinical judgment the therapist makes based on the examination. The evaluation results in the determination of the diagnosis, prognosis, and interventions. The *diagnosis is both the process and the end result of evaluating the examination data.* The *prognosis* is a judgment about the level of optimal improvement the patient may attain and the amount of time needed to reach that level. *Interventions* are the skilled techniques and activities that make up the treatment plan.[12]

Types and Content of Examinations and Evaluations

The PT should always perform an initial examination and evaluation and a discharge examination and evaluation of the patient and may perform one or more interim evaluations, depending on the length of time the patient is receiving physical therapy care. The PT follows the APTA's *Guidelines for Physical Therapy Documentation*[13] outlining the recommended content of the reports. These Guidelines are included in Appendix D of this textbook. A description of each type of examination/evaluation report follows this discussion with a list of the recommended information contained in the report. The medical record content categories discussed in this chapter are indicated in bold next to the physical therapy examination and evaluation information appropriate for each category to demonstrate how the physical therapy report conforms to the documentation content in the medical record.

SUMMARY

The information documented in the medical record consists of the following:

1. Problems that require medical attention
2. Data relevant to the patient's medical/physical therapy diagnosis
3. A treatment plan to address the problems
4. Goals of the treatment plan
5. A record of the administration of the treatments
6. Results or effectiveness of the treatment plan

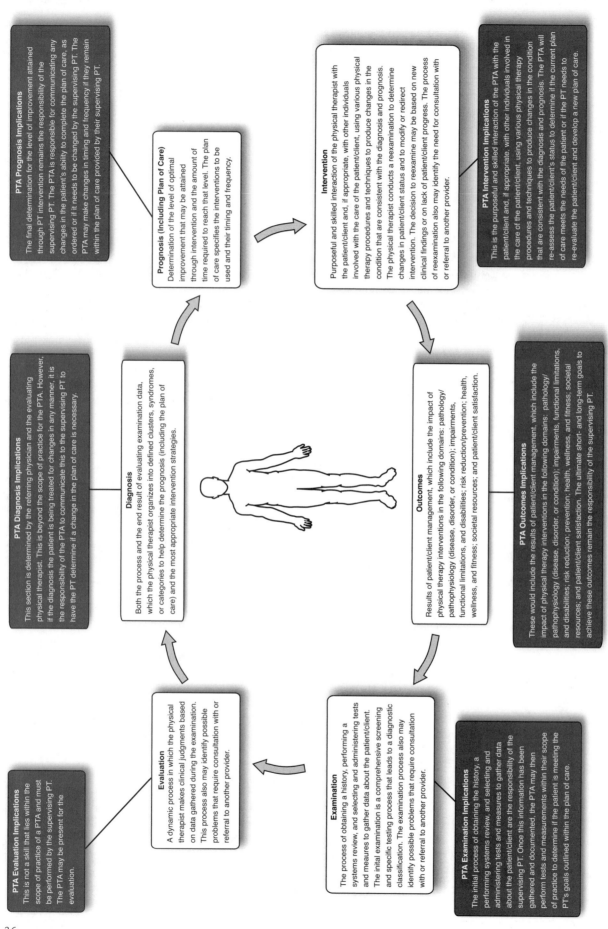

PTA Prognosis Implications

The final determination for the level of improvement attained through PT intervention remains the responsibility of the supervising PT. The PTA is responsible for communicating any changes in the patient's ability to complete the plan of care, as ordered or if it needs to be changed by the supervising PT. The PTA may make changes in timing and frequency if they remain within the plan of care provided by their supervising PT.

Prognosis (Including Plan of Care)

Determination of the level of optimal improvement that may be attained through intervention and the amount of time required to reach that level. The plan of care specifies the interventions to be used and their timing and frequency.

Intervention

Purposeful and skilled interaction of the physical therapist with the patient/client and, if appropriate, with other individuals involved with the care of the patient/client, using various physical therapy procedures and techniques to produce changes in the condition that are consistent with the diagnosis and prognosis. The physical therapist conducts a reexamination to determine changes in patient/client status and to modify or redirect intervention. The decision to reexamine may be based on new clinical findings or on lack of patient/client progress. The process of reexamination also may identify the need for consultation with or referral to another provider.

PTA Intervention Implications

This is the purposeful and skilled interaction of the PTA with the patient/client and, if appropriate, with other individuals involved in the care of the patient/client, using various physical therapy procedures and techniques to produce changes in the condition that are consistent with the diagnosis and prognosis. The PTA will re-assess the patient/client's status to determine if the current plan of care meets the needs of the patient or if the PT needs to re-evaluate the patient/client and develop a new plan of care.

PTA Diagnosis Implications

This section is determined by the referring physician and the evaluating physical therapist. This is beyond the scope of practice for the PTA. However, if the diagnosis the patient is being treated for changes in any manner, it is the responsibility of the PTA to communicate this to the supervising PT to have the PT determine if a change in the plan of care is necessary.

Diagnosis

Both the process and the end result of evaluating examination data, which the physical therapist organizes into defined clusters, syndromes, or categories to help determine the prognosis (including the plan of care) and the most appropriate intervention strategies.

Outcomes

Results of patient/client management, which include the impact of physical therapy interventions in the following domains: pathology/pathophysiology (disease, disorder, or condition); impairments, functional limitations, and disabilities; risk reduction/prevention; health, wellness, and fitness; societal resources; and patient/client satisfaction.

PTA Outcomes Implications

These would include the results of patient/client management, which include the impact of physical therapy interventions in the following domains: pathology/pathophysiology (disease, disorder, or condition); impairments, functional limitations, and disabilities; risk reduction; prevention; health, wellness, and fitness; societal resources; and patient/client satisfaction. The ultimate short- and long-term goals to achieve these outcomes remain the responsibility of the supervising PT.

PTA Evaluation Implications

This is not a skill that lies within the scope of practice of a PTA and must be performed by the supervising PT. The PTA may be present for the evaluation.

Evaluation

A dynamic process in which the physical therapist makes clinical judgments based on data gathered during the examination. This process also may identify possible problems that require consultation with or referral to another provider.

Examination

The process of obtaining a history, performing a systems review, and selecting and administering tests and measures to gather data about the patient/client. The initial examination is a comprehensive screening and specific testing process that leads to a diagnostic classification. The examination process also may identify possible problems that require consultation with or referral to another provider.

PTA Examination Implications

The initial process of obtaining the history, performing systems review, and selecting and administering tests and measures to gather data about the patient/client are the responsibility of the supervising PT. Once this information has been gathered and documented, the PTA may then perform tests and measurements within their scope of practice to determine if the patient is meeting the PT's goals outlined within the plan of care.

Figure 2—13 Treatment responsibilities of the PT versus the PTA. (Adapted from American Physical Therapy Association. (2003 June). *Guide to physical therapist practice* (ed. 2, p. 35), with permission.)

The documentation content describes the medical care from the moment the patient is first seen by the medical professional. The information reporting the effectiveness of the treatment is the content used to determine the quality of the care provided, measure outcomes, research the most effective treatment procedures, and determine reimbursement.

A comparison of the medical diagnosis with the physical therapy diagnosis was presented. The physical therapy diagnosis is the identification of the abnormalities and dysfunctions (impairments) causing a functional limitation. The functional limitation is the primary reason the patient seeks physical therapy, and improvement of this limitation is the goal of physical therapy treatment.

Information about treatment procedures (e.g., their purposes, expected results, and any possible risks or side effects) must be explained to the patient or a representative of the patient. He or she must agree to the treatment plan before it is started. This agreement, called *informed consent,* is often made official by the patient's signing an informed consent form, which is placed in the medical record.

The documentation content is found in the written evaluation reports and the progress notes. The PT performs and writes initial, interim, and discharge examination/evaluation reports. The PTA can assist the PT in the examination but does not evaluate. The PTA documents the progress notes, which is the focus of this book.

*The Guide to Physical Therapist Practice is a publication by The American Physical Therapy Association and describes the following: (1) physical therapists and their roles in health care; (2) the generally accepted elements of physical therapy patient/client management; (3) the types of tests and measurements used by physical therapists; (4) the types of interventions physical therapists use; (5) the anticipated goals of the interventions; and (6) the expected outcomes of physical therapy patient/client management. Preferred practice patterns are descriptions about common physical therapy management strategies for specific diagnostic groups. The patterns serve as a guide for the physical therapist when planning comprehensive plans of care.[10]

REFERENCES

1. *Rehabilitation documentation software.* Accessed on March 2, 2007 from http://www.rehabdocumentation.com.
2. *TheraClin Systems documentation software.* Accessed on March 2, 2007 from http://www.theraclin.com.
3. *Clinicient Insight software.* Accessed on March 2, 2007 from http://www.clinicient.com.
4. *TheraSourse documentation software.* Accessed on March 2, 2007 from http://www.TheraSourse.com.
5. Martin, K. D. (1990). Individualized educational program and individualized family service plan. *Physical therapy practice in educational environments: Policies and guidelines* (p. 6.1). Alexandria, VA: APTA.
6. Centers for Medicare and Medicaid Services. Accessed on March 2, 2007 from http://www.cms.hhs.gov/center/hospital.asp.
7. Swanson, G. (December 1995). *Essentials for the future of physical therapy, every therapist's concern.* A continuing education course. Duluth, MN: Minnesota Chapter, American Physical Therapy Association.
8. Scott, R. W. (2006). *Legal aspects of documenting patient care,* Gaithersburg, MD: Aspen.
9. El-Din, D., & Smith, G. J. (February 1995). *Performance based documentation: A tool for functional documentation.* Reno, NV: APTA.
10. American Physical Therapy Association. (June 2003). *The guide to physical therapist practice.* Alexandria, VA: APTA.
11. World Health Organization. (2001). *International classification of functioning, disability, and health.* Geneva, Switzerland.
12. American Physical Therapy Association. Content, development and concepts. In *The guide to physical therapist practice.* Alexandria, VA: APTA.
12a. World Health Organization. (2001). *International classification of functioning, disability, and health.* Geneva, Switzerland.
13. Sahrmann, S. A. (1988). Diagnosis by physical therapist—a prerequisite for treatment. A special communication. *Physical Therapy, 68,* 1703–1786.

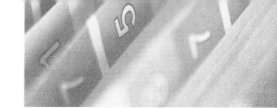

Review Exercises

1. List the **six** categories of documentation content, and describe the content of each category.

2. Explain the difference between **source-oriented** and **problem-oriented** documentation.

3. Define a **functional** limitation.

4. Compare and contrast the **medical** diagnosis and the **physical therapy** diagnosis.

5. **Define** PSPG, DEP, and FOR.

6. List **three** formats in which documentation content may be presented, and identify the **types** of physical therapy facilities most likely to use each format.

7. What is an **impairment?** Give **three** examples.

Practice Exercise 1 ➤ *You read in the PT's initial evaluation that your patient has a fractured right femur that has healed. He is left with 2/5 strength (normal strength is 5/5) in the quadriceps and is unable to transfer independently in and out of bed or a chair.*

What is the medical problem? _____

What is the abnormality or dysfunction of the musculoskeletal system?

_____

What is the functional limitation? _____

_____

Practice Exercise 2 ➤ *You read in the PT's evaluation that your patient has had a cerebral vascular accident (e.g., stroke) and now has difficulty moving his left arm and leg. The PT states that the patient has weakness and extensor hypertonus in his left lower extremity with inability to ambulate stairs independently.*

What is the medical diagnosis? (pathology) _____

What is the abnormality or dysfunction of the neuromuscular system (impairment)?

_____

What is the functional limitation? _____

Practice Exercise 3 ➤ *You read in the PT's evaluation that your patient has an incomplete spinal cord injury causing lower extremity paraparesis and an inability to stand.*

What is the medical diagnosis? (pathology) _____

What is the impairment? _____

What is the functional limitation? _____

Practice Exercise 4 ➤ *Identify the documentation responsibilities of the PT and the PTA. Place "PT" next to the items that are a responsibility of the PT only. Place "PTA" next to items that are documentation tasks for the PTA.*

_____ Initial examination and evaluation

_____ Discharge examination and evaluation

_____ Progress notes

_____ Change in treatment plan

_____ Reexamination and reevaluation

Practice Exercise 5 ➤ *Identify the pathology, impairment, functional limitation, and disability after each patient description.*

1. Mr. Jones, a professional football player, will never be able to play football again because he fractured a vertebra and severed his spinal cord. His legs are paralyzed and he cannot stand or walk.

   Pathology _____

   Impairment _____

Functional limitation _____

Disability _____

2. Sally received third-degree burns on both hands, and the scar tissue causes limited ROM in her fingers and wrists. She is unable to pick up or manipulate small objects, so she is unable to return to any work that requires fine hand manipulation.

Pathology _____

Impairment _____

Functional limitation _____

Disability _____

3. Mrs. Williams has rheumatoid arthritis with limited ROM in both knees and hips. She is unable to climb stairs or steps, so she must live and function in an environment that has no stairs or steps.

Pathology _____

Impairment _____

Functional limitation _____

Disability _____

4. Mr. Nelson's left leg was crushed in a motor vehicle accident. His leg was amputated just above his knee. He does not have the muscle strength to walk with his prosthesis (artificial leg) without the help of a cane. He will not be able to return to his old job as a railroad brakeman.

Pathology _____

Impairment _____

Functional limitation _____

Disability _____

5. Joe received a head injury in a snowmobile accident. He now has difficulty maintaining his balance when walking and frequently feels dizzy. He walks with a wheeled walker and always needs someone nearby, in case he feels dizzy while walking.

Pathology _____

Impairment _____

Functional limitation _____

Disability _____

6. A little girl in the third grade has spina bifida, which has caused her legs to be very weak. She can walk independently with crutches, but she cannot maintain her balance when she tries to open doors.

Pathology _____

Impairment _____

Functional limitation _____

Disability _____

Practice Exercise 6 ➤ *You are a PTA working on the orthopedic floor at the local hospital. You are treating Earl, a 62-year-old farmer, who has just had Ⓡ total knee arthroplasty surgery. The PT saw him on day one, postoperation. The discharge goals are (1) independent ambulation on tiling, carpeting, stairs, and inclines with the least restrictive and most appropriate assistive device; and (2) independent transfers. Active knee ROM should be 90° at discharge. Treatments are to include CPM, 1 hr on/1 hr off until 70° is reached; isometric exercises for quads, gluts, hamstrings; ankle pumps; TKE; SLR; and active knee flexion. Gait training is to start on day one in the a.m. A cold/ice pack may be used on the knee as needed.*

Document the following treatment sessions on the following flow sheet.

Day 2: All isometric exercises independent with good coordination. CPM increased to 40°. Active knee flexion while supine 3°–30°. Bed mobility transfers (supine to sit) mod. assist of one to support knee. Unable to do SLR independently. In sitting, still requires support to Ⓡ aknee as pain too severe for initiation of ROM exercises. Ice pack to knee almost continuous. Drain in place for a.m. session; removed by p.m. session. Able to stand at side of bed, PWB RLE. Did not attempt ambulation because of pain.

Day 3: A.M.: Able to sit at side of bed with AROM to 45°, much pain. BP 140/85 mm Hg, pulse at 72 BPM before standing. Stood at side of bed with mod. assist of one, PWB to approx. 50% of body weight on RLE, used walker. Took several steps to chair, then sat. Uses standing pivot transfer with walker. BP 145/88 mm Hg, pulse 100 BPM. Independent with all exercises. Supine knee flexion to 35°. CPM to 60° p.m. as in a.m., but able to ambulate 50 ft 1X with walker, PWB at 50% body weight. Continues to keep ice pack on knee.

Day 4: A.M.: Ambulated 50 ft 2X with walker on level surface, tile, and carpet. Sitting AROM 60°, CPM increased to 70°. Supine AROM 5°–55° flexion. Min. assist with SLR. P.M.: Ambulated 50 ft 2X with walker, SBA. Ambulated 60 ft 1X with crutches on level, min. assist of one. Remains PWB with up to 75% body weight. AROM sitting to 75°, supine 5°–60°. SBA for supine to sit transfer, independent transfer sit to stand. Independent with SLR. Ice pack discontinued this morning.

Day 5: A.M.: Independent with all exercises and all standing pivot transfers. CPM discontinued last night by nursing. Ambulates independently 125 ft with crutches, 3-point step through gait on tile and carpeting. SBA on stairs and inclines. Knee ROM sitting to 85°, supine 5°–80°. PT to see patient in P.M. for discharge evaluation.

TOTAL KNEE ARTHROPLASTY

	Date 8-8-06		Date		Date		Date		Date	
	am	pm	am	pm	am	pm	am	pm	am	pm
CPM Degrees	25									
CPM Time	1 hr on/1 hr off									
Knee ROM AA = Active Assist A = Active Supine										
Sitting										
Exercises: Isometrics Quads/Gluts/HS										
Ankle Pumps										
TKE										
SLR										
Active Knee Flex										
Transfers: Bed Mobility										
Toilet/Commode										
Shower Seat										
Car Transfer										
Standing Pivot										
Sliding Board										
Supine <- -> Sit										
Sit <- -> Stand										
Balance: Sitting										
Standing										
Ambulation: Device										
Weight Bearing										
Pattern										
Distance										
Surface										
Assist										
Stairs										
Blood Pressure										
Pulse										
Modalities	Ice pack prn									
THERAPIST	Jennifer Nice, PT									

PHYSICAL THERAPY PROGRESS

PRECAUTIONS: Drain in place 8-8-06

NAME: Earl

Practice Exercise 7 ➤   *Place MD by the medical diagnoses, IMP by the impairments, and FL by the functional limitations.*

_____ 1. Diabetes

_____ 2. Rhomboid strength 3/5

_____ 3. Instability

_____ 4. Unable to reach top of head

_____ 5. Multiple sclerosis

_____ 6. Fractured neck of the femur

_____ 7. Inability to walk one block

_____ 8. Cannot sleep more than 3 hours

_____ 9. Frequent falling

_____ 10. Paralysis

_____ 11. Severed ulnar nerve

_____ 12. 10°–90° knee flexion

_____ 13. Cerebral palsy

_____ 14. Hypermobility

_____ 15. Unable to sit unsupported

_____ 16. Circumducted gait pattern

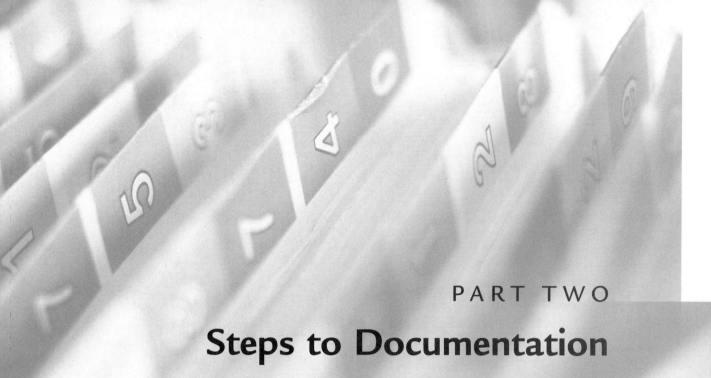

PART TWO

Steps to Documentation

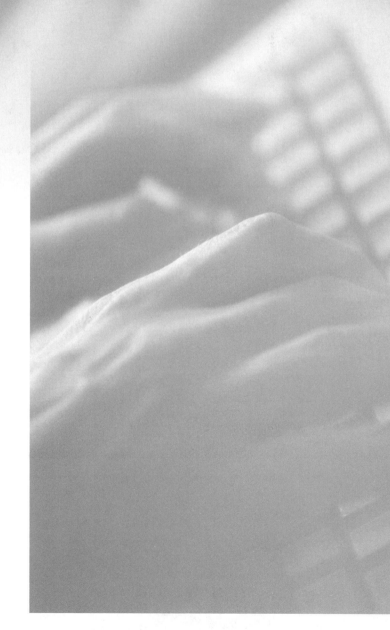

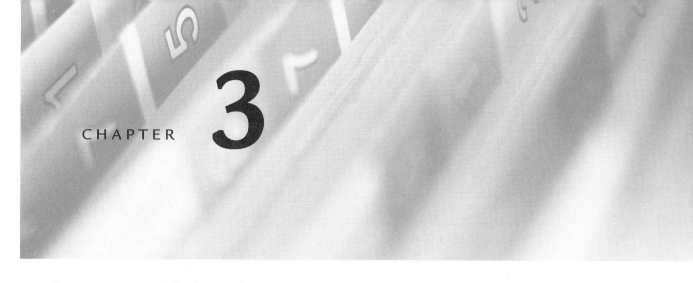

CHAPTER 3

What Is Subjective Data and Why It Is Important

LEARNING OBJECTIVES

After studying this chapter, the student will be able to:
☐ Use "person first" terminology.
☐ Differentiate between subjective and objective data.
☐ Explain the difference between examination, evaluation, and discharge.
☐ Identify the basic information included in the summation of care.
☐ Compare and contrast documentation responsibilities between the PT and the PTA.
☐ Select relevant subjective data to document the patient's physical therapy diagnosis and treatment.
☐ Identify common characteristics of good listening skills.
☐ Organize subjective data for easy reading and understanding.
☐ Demonstrate adherence to the recommended guidelines for documenting subjective data.
☐ Use appropriate methods to properly document information about the patient's pain.

INTRODUCTION

The subjective data, "S," is the information that the patient or family member tells the therapist. Information in the medical record communicates the story of a patient's medical care. This format is used to organize information within the patient's chart and varies from facility to facility. In addition, the appearance of the chart depends on the type of clinical facility. For example, a hospital medical record is different from the record format used in a physical therapy private practice office. The student PTA during his or her clinical experience or the newly employed therapist should become familiar with the facility's medical record format from the very beginning; the record is a good communication tool only if the reader knows where to find the information.

In addition, it is important for the PTA student and newly employed therapist to be able to organize their thoughts into a succinct account of the treatment session with the patient once the PT has completed the evaluation and developed the plan of care. For that reason, the SOAP note provides an excellent medium for learning how to put information related to the patient in an outline type format. In this manner, the PTA student is able to develop the necessary skills to communicate how the patient is progressing, assess problems that may develop during the treatment session, develop time frames for progression within the plan of care, make discharge recommendations, and make recommendations for other health-care treatments.

Person First Language

Any documentation should address information related to a patient in "person first language." The meaning of this statement relates to the person and the disabling characteristic for which the individual is receiving medical treatment. The disability should not define the person; instead, emphasis should be placed on the person's identity, not their physical limitations. Terms that follow are examples of words or expressions to be avoided:

- The paralyzed patient
- The hemiplegic patient
- CVAs
- Amputees
- The CVA patient
- The paraplegic student

Instead, use words or expressions similar to those in the following list:

- The male patient with a T12 spinal cord injury
- The person who is disabled
- The woman who has had a CVA
- Mr. Jones, who is paralyzed
- Mrs. Smith, a 62-year-old woman with spina bifida[1]

DOCUMENTATION SPECIFICS

In addition to the basic sections of a SOAP note, other identifying information should be included in the medical record of a patient receiving physical therapy services. (Fig. 3–1) These include the information gathered in the PT evaluation completed in the first session with the patient. This evaluation will also include the patient's plan of care. The PTA will continue to follow this initial plan of care and assess the patient's progress, as reported to the PT. Through this reporting process, the PTA should communicate the need for a change in the plan of care because the patient goals have or have not been met, the need to progress the patient, or the need to develop a discharge plan. The PTA is not responsible for determining when to discharge the patient but is responsible for communicating the patient's progression toward a preparation for discharge. Within the evaluation, reassessment, and discharge notes, the following information may be included.

Initial Examination and Evaluation

The initial examination and evaluation are performed the first time the PT meets with the patient. This written report contains the following information:

1. *History, observations, and risk factor identification.* General statistics about the patient are obtained before the evaluation is performed. Some of this information may be found elsewhere in the chart, such as in the notes from admissions, the emergency room, or the physician. Examples are age, medical diagnosis, name, sex, date of birth, physician, complications, and precautions. All these data are required in the medical record, but all may not be in the PT's evaluation if they are already located elsewhere in the chart.

2. *Component identification.* Components of an evaluation should include information about the following:
   a. Strength
   b. Active and passive ROM
   c. Functional abilities
   d. Pain level
   e. Presence of abnormal muscle tone
   f. Ability to communicate and understand simple commands
   g. Need for adaptive equipment
   h. Presence of automatic reactions
   i. Presence of any abnormal reflex patterns
   j. Level of independence in daily care
3. *Subjective data:* Information obtained from what the patient tells the PT or PTA during the interview. Examples are the onset of injury/disease/pain, chief complaint, location of complaints, functional limitations, home situation, lifestyle, goals, and pertinent medical history.
4. *Objective data:* Results of objective testing and observations of the patient. Examples are physical status, such as strength, endurance, skin condition, ROM, and neurologic status; functional status, such as mobility, transfers, ambulation, activities of daily living, and abilities at work/school/home; mental status, such as cognition, orientation, communication problems, judgment, and ability to follow directions; status of appropriate reflex responses such as presence of primitive and automatic reactions; status of muscles and alignment to include muscle tone and symmetrical alignment; functional abilities such as the level of function, and the need for any assistive devices.
5. *Evaluation:* PT's interpretation of the results of the testing and observations.
6. *Diagnosis:* The physical therapy diagnosis identifying the impairments and functional limitations.
7. *Goals:* Anticipated goals and expected outcomes related to resolving the diagnosis, written in measurable and functional terms.
8. *Treatment plan or recommendation:* Treatment plans related to accomplishing the goals, including specific interventions, their frequency and duration, a statement regarding the prognosis (the patient's rehabilitation potential or expectations of treatment effectiveness), an estimate of the length of time the patient will be receiving physical therapy treatment, and a schedule or plan for evaluating the effectiveness of the treatment.
9. *Physical therapist designation:* Authentication and appropriate designation of the physical therapist, including signature, title, and professional license number.

Reexamination and Reevaluation

Documentation of the continuum of physical therapy care that the patient is receiving is recorded by the PT in the reexamination and reevaluation reports and by the PTA or PT in the progress notes. The content of the PT's reexamination and reevaluation reports is discussed in this chapter, and because it is the purpose of this textbook, the content of the progress note is discussed in the remaining chapters.

Interim or progress examinations and evaluations are performed by the PT periodically throughout the period the patient is receiving physical therapy. The progress examination and evaluation content includes the following information:

1. *Intervention or service provided:* Treatment procedures administered, involving a summary of the interventions and other services provided by the PT or PTA since the initial evaluation.
2. *Patient status, progress, or regression:* Subjective data—Patient's subjective information as to the effectiveness of the interventions. Objective data—A repeat of the testing and observations made in the initial examination.
3. *Reexamination and reevaluation:* Results or effectiveness of the treatment plan, including the following:

The PTA becomes familiar with the patient's medical record by reading the PT's initial examination/evaluation report and the initial evaluation reports of the physician and any other health-care providers treating the patient. During treatment sessions, the PTA should listen for any information that relates to treatment effectiveness and accomplishment of goals and outcomes. The PTA should also report to the PT and document in the progress note any information heard that is not in the record but may be important for effective and quality physical therapy care of the patient.

Medical History

INITIAL EXAMINATION: Information about the patient's previous medical conditions and treatments are in the medical history section of the medical chart and in the initial examination reports.

PROGRESS NOTE: Listen for any medical history information that was not reported earlier but is relevant to the patient's treatment and record such information in the progress note.

Example: Sue, the PTA, sneezes four times as she escorts Mrs. Smith to the treatment cubicle to prepare for an ultrasound treatment. As she excuses herself to go wash her hands, Sue explains that she is not sick but is allergic to pollen during this time of the year. Mrs. Smith mentions her allergy to a perfume that Sue knows is in the ultrasound gel. As Sue positions Mrs. Smith on the plinth, Mrs. Smith states that she itched for a while "right where the PT gave my first ultrasound treatment yesterday." Sue makes a mental note to use ultrasound lotion instead of the gel today, to inform the PT, and be sure to document this in the progress note. Figure 3–3 demonstrates how this information is included in the progress note.

Environment: Lifestyle, Home Situation, Work Tasks, School Needs, and Leisure Activities

INITIAL EXAMINATION: The PT or PTA has already interviewed the patient to learn about his or her needs at home, school, or work to help plan treatment goals.

PROGRESS NOTE: Listen for any further information that will influence treatment and document it in the progress note.

Example: Sue knows from reading the medical record that her patient, Harry, has a toilet next to a combination tub and shower with grab bars at home, and that his bathroom is small. Harry had a stroke, and his balance is slightly unsteady. Sue is planning to teach him to slide from the toilet onto the edge of the tub, swing his feet into the tub, then stand for his shower. Today, during his treatment session, Harry's wife comments that her back is aching because she just spent an hour cleaning the shower doors and the track in which the doors slide. "That track is uncomfortable to sit on," thought Sue. "I need to think of a better method for Harry to transfer into his tub."

Emotions or Attitudes

INITIAL EXAMINATION: The PT or PTA records the patient's attitude or emotional state presented at the time of the examination.

PROGRESS NOTE: Patient's attitudes can change during the course of treatment, or they might not have presented their true feelings to the PT during the initial examination. The PTA needs to be alert for these changes.

Example: PTA Jim treats his patient Sam, who had a stroke. Yesterday, they worked on balance and stability using the hands-and-knees position and batting a balloon while in sitting position. Today Sam refuses to go to physical therapy. He states that he does not want to play children's games and that if he could just go home, he would be fine. Jim realizes he needs to consult the PT and restructure the treatment sessions to work on balance and stability in activities Sam will want to be doing at home.

Goals or Functional Outcomes

Goals or functional outcomes are set by the patient and the PT during the initial evaluation.

PROGRESS NOTE: Goals may need to be modified as the patient and the PTA become better acquainted and the PTA learns more about the patient's needs and desires.

Example: Sam told the PT that he needs to be able to climb only two steps to get into his house; the rest of his house is on one floor. They set a stair-climbing goal: "To be able to climb two steps independently using the railing on the left and be able to ascend and descend a curb independently with no ambulation device." One week later, during a treatment session, Sam is telling Jim about his cabin on a nearby lake and how anxious he is to go to the cabin and go fishing. Sam casually mentions that there are six wooden steps down to the dock. Jim makes a mental note to share this information with the PT and to suggest that the goal be modified.

Figure 3–1   Examples of information included in a SOAP note.

Unusual Events or Chief Complaints

GOALS AND OUTCOMES: Chief complaints are the patient's symptoms of the disease or dysfunction requiring treatment.

PROGRESS NOTE: During treatment sessions, reports of unusual events may indicate a physiological change in the patient, or may be evidence of the effectiveness or ineffectiveness of the treatment. Reports may also indicate the patient's compliance and other health conditions encountered during the week.

Example 1: Patient states she did not do her home exercises this week because she had the flu. The PTA will realize that this may be why the patient hasn't progressed this week and that this is relevant information for the subjective data in the progress note.

Example 2: PTA Brenda treats Ray, who has a spinal cord injury. Today she goes to Ray's hospital room to take him to physical therapy. Ray complains he is feeling weak, has chills, and is somewhat light-headed. He doesn't think he can exercise in therapy today. Brenda talks with Ray's nurse and cancels this morning's therapy, writing about Ray's complaints and her conversation with Ray's nurse in the progress notes. Brenda checks on Ray in the afternoon, and he tells her that he has a urinary tract infection and is just now starting the medication. He still feels weak and light-headed. Brenda cancels the afternoon treatment session, describing Ray's complaints in the subjective area of the progress note.

Response to Treatment

Reporting the patient's response documents the effectiveness of treatment and influences future treatment plans.

Example: PTA Brenda treats Robert, who has a mild lumbar disc protrusion and complains of waking up often in the night with tingling in his left leg. During yesterday's treatment session, Brenda showed Robert how to use pillows and a rolled towel to support his spine and maintain proper positioning while sleeping. Today, Robert reports that he awoke only three times last night because of back soreness and didn't have any tingling in his leg. Brenda makes a mental note to quote Robert in the subjective section of the progress note to provide evidence that her instructions in sleeping positions were effective.

Level of Functioning

The initial examination describes the patient's functional level at the time of the examination.

PROGRESS NOTE: The patient's description of his or her functional level may help the PTA assess the patient's progress or response to treatment.

Example: PTA Mary is treating Mr. Jones, who had an acute flare-up of osteoarthritis in his hands. His chief complaint during the initial evaluation was inability to dress himself, especially handling buttons and snaps, because of the pain. Today he arrives wearing a sweater, which he said he buttoned without needing to ask for help. This comment may be evidence in the progress note that Mr. Jones has met a goal or outcome.

Figure 3–1   (Continued)

a. Interpretation of objective test results and observations and a comparison with data from the initial evaluation
b. Statement addressing the accomplishment of the goals set in the initial evaluation and any new goals set
c. Information regarding any change in the patient's status
d. Treatment plan written by the PT indicating whether the initial plan is to be continued or changed
e. Signature, title, and license number of the physical therapist

Summation of Care   This discharge examination and evaluation is the patient's final evaluation and the final note about the patient in the medical record. **This note must be written by the supervising PT.** A properly written discharge note follows the APTA's guidelines and should include the following information:

1. Brief summary of the treatment that was provided (intervention procedures administered)
2. Relevant information provided by the patient (subjective data)
3. Interpretation of repeated testing and observations and a comparison with data from the latest interim evaluation or initial evaluation (objective data and results or effectiveness of interventions)

4. Statement regarding the accomplishment of anticipated goals and expected outcomes (results or effectiveness of the treatment plan)
5. Further interventions or care needed after discharge
6. Plans for follow up or monitoring after discharge
7. Signature, title, and professional license number of the PT[2]

Discharge Notes

Physical therapy professionals disagree about the definitions of *discharge evaluation* and *discharge summary*. Some believe the evaluation and the summary are the same, whereas others consider them different types of documents.

If a discharge summary is considered the same as a discharge evaluation, then the evaluation/summary will have content that interprets the test results and identifies the plans for the patient after discharge. Decisions about the patient's care after discharge may be made based on the information in the discharge evaluation/summary. In this case, only a PT can write a discharge summary.

When a patient's treatment has been discontinued, the PTA may write the discharge summary or note. This note only **summarizes** the care given the patient and the patient's response to the interventions and objectively states the functional status of the patient at the time of discharge. There can be *no interpretation of the data or evaluation of the patient's status*, the PTA can make no plan for the patient's care after discharge is identified, and no decisions can be made based on changes in the plan of care. If the PTA writes a discharge summary of this nature, there still must be a discharge evaluation written by the PT as the final note in the patient's medical record. In any situation, the *final documentation in the patient's physical therapy chart must be written by the PT*[2].

PTA Involvement

Although the PTA does not perform evaluations, he or she may assist the PT with the examination procedures. The PTA may take notes and help gather the subjective data. The PTA also may take measurements, perform some tests, and record the results. However, the PTA may not interpret the results. Performing the tests and recording the results constitute *data collection*. Interpreting the results involves making a judgment about their value. This is called *evaluating*. Examples of tests and measurements that are part of a PTA's data collection skills are girth measurements, manual muscle testing of muscle groups, goniometry measurements, and vital signs.

During the course of a patient's treatment, the PTA is often expected to repeat the measurements and tests to record the patient's progress since the initial examination and evaluation. These objective data are more reliable when the same person performs the tests and measurements in a consistent manner throughout the course of the patient's treatment. In addition, assisting the PT with the examination offers the PTA and patient an opportunity to become acquainted so the patient will feel comfortable working with the PTA as the treatment plan is carried out.

When writing progress notes, the PTA refers to the problems, goals and outcomes, and treatment plans in the initial and interim evaluation reports. Progress notes should record the effectiveness of the treatment plan by comparing the patient's progress toward accomplishing the goals and outcomes with the status of the patient at the initial evaluation.

Documentation Responsibilities

The documentation content is found in the examination and evaluation reports and progress notes. The PT is responsible for the evaluations, consultations, and decision-making required for the patient's physical therapy health care. Therefore, the PT's documentation responsibilities are to record the following information:

1. Initial evaluation, which includes the goals and outcomes and the treatment plan
2. Interim or progress evaluations performed
3. Changes in the treatment plan
4. Discharge information[2]

The PT may also write progress notes. The primary documentation responsibility of the PTA is to record the progress or interim notes.

The PTA must be familiar with the content of the PT's examination and evaluation reports. The reports inform the PTA of the patient's medical and physical therapy diagnoses. The PTA follows the treatment plan outlined in the evaluations and directs all treatment sessions toward accomplishing the goals and outcomes listed in the evaluations.

GENERAL SOAP NOTE DATA

Information gathered about a patient may include both subjective and objective data. Most of this information is gathered at the time of admission or the first time the patient is seen by each medical service provider. However, information is being gathered continuously throughout the span of the patient's care. Data gathered when the patient is admitted will be located in the reports of the initial examinations performed by the various medical services. For example, a young male student is admitted to the emergency room (ER) at Community Hospital at 2:45 a.m. on Saturday after being involved in a motorcycle accident. Information is gathered when the patient is admitted to the ER, when the patient is taken to radiology, when the patient is admitted to the orthopedic unit, and when laboratory tests are performed. More information will be gathered when the patient is first seen by physical therapy, occupational therapy, and social services. Examples of the data gathered by each discipline are highlighted in Table 2–1 of Chapter 2.

For further delineation of patient information, the PT and PTA can report the information in a SOAP note format. This type of format helps the beginning therapist organize patient information pertinent to the treatment session. It includes a subjective data, objective data, assessment, and plan sections. A **general** explanation of each section of the SOAP note follows:

Subjective Data

Information **told** to the health-care provider comprises subjective data. Subjective data include:

1. Information about the patient's past medical history
2. Symptoms or complaints that caused the patient to seek medical attention
3. Factors that produced the symptoms
4. The patient's functional and lifestyle needs
5. The patient's goals or expectations about medical care

Typically, data relevant to the patient's condition and reason for admission are obtained by interviewing the patient or significant others. Collecting subjective data is an ongoing process while medical care is being provided. The information reflects the patient's response to treatment and the effectiveness of treatment.

The PT and PTA seek information provided by the patient. The PT documents subjective data in the physical therapy examination and evaluation reports. The PTA documents subjective data in the daily or weekly progress notes. Regardless of the organizational format used, subjective data content in the physical therapy examination and evaluation report and the progress note is typically located at the beginning of or early in the note. For example, it is recorded in the S section of the SOAP outline, in the D section of the DEP format, and in the F section of the FOR. Subjective data content is included in the S (status) section of the PSPG organization.

Subjective data are critically important in physical therapy examination and evaluation reports. As part of the continuum of care in progress notes, subjective data provide evidence of treatment effectiveness or progress toward the functional goals.

Objective Data

Objective information includes information that is *reproducible and readily demonstrable*, gathered by carefully examining the patient by using data-collecting methods such as measurements, tests, and observations. These methods can be **reproduced** by any medical professional with the same training as the one who first performed the examination.

Objective data are the signs of the patient's condition. Reviewing the signs by repeating the measurements, tests, and observations is also an ongoing process for determining treatment effectiveness and patient progress. The PT performs the physical therapy examination/evaluation and uses objective methods to gather data. These data are used to determine the physical therapy diagnosis. The PTA repeats any measurements, tests, and observations within the scope of his or her practice to determine the patient's progress toward accomplishing the treatment goals.

Assessment   Assessment is a summary of the subjective and objective information. In this section, the PT interprets, makes a clinical judgment, and sets functional outcomes and goals based on the information in the subjective and objective sections of the SOAP note. The PTA summarizes the information described in the two preceding sections and reports the progress being made toward accomplishing the goals.

Plan   The plan describes what will happen next. The PTA describes what he or she may need to do before or during the next treatment session or what the patient or caregivers may need to do.

Subjective Information   The S section contains the subjective data; that is, information provided by the patient, his or her caregiver, a family member, or significant other. Each time the patient is seen, he or she is interviewed and questioned. This information is gathered, and these symptoms of the patient's disease or dysfunction are **described** in the subjective section.

Examples of SOAP Note Organization   Suppose your 10-year-old daughter has been diagnosed by your doctor as having strep throat and an ear infection. You obtained medication and have started her on the treatment. It is the next morning.

> **5-18-06: Dx/Pr:**   Strep throat and ear infection.
>
> ---
>
> **S:**   Pt. reports pain in Ⓡ ear, feels too tired to go to school.
>
> **O:**   Temperature 100.8°F, down 2° from last night, skin color pale. Pt. sat at breakfast table 20 min before needing to lie down and was not able to eat solid food. Pt. took medication, 2 tablets, 8:00 a.m. per instructions.
>
> **A:**   Pt.'s fever decreasing but temp. not at goal of 98.6°F. Pt. is not able to stay up all day for school and is not able to consume a normal diet.
>
> **P:**   Will call attendance office to excuse pt. from school; will continue medication per Dr.'s orders.
>
> —Super Parent, PTA

Here's another example. You are a PTA teaching a patient to walk with crutches. This patient had a skiing accident that resulted in multiple fractures of bones in the ankle joint. The ankle has been surgically treated and placed in a cast, and the patient is not permitted to bear weight on the foot.

> **2-16-06: Dx:**   Fractured Ⓛ ankle repaired and casted.
> **Pr:**   No weight-bearing on Ⓛ leg, requiring ambulation with crutches.
>
> ---
>
> **S:**   Pt. states he plans to go home tomorrow and needs to climb a flight of stairs in his house and to manage ramps and curbs to return to work.
>
> **O:**   After 3 trials requiring standby assist for sense of security and verbal cueing, patient independently ascended and descended a flight of 12 stairs by using the railing (up on Ⓡ, down on Ⓛ) and axillary crutches, NWB on Ⓛ, and independently managed a ramp and four curbs of various heights. Pt. independently transferred in and out of his car, accurately following instructions.
>
> **A:**   Pt. accomplished outcome of being able to independently manage stairs, ramps, and curbs for functioning within his house and for ambulating in the community for return to work. Will recommend discharge to PT because all goals have been met and pt. is at his highest functional level.
>
> **P:**   Will arrange for PT's discharge evaluation tomorrow.
>
> —Alice Assistant, PTA

You can see how thinking *SOAP* **organizes** information so it can be documented in a logical sequence. This organization also makes it easy to find information.

Criticism of SOAP Notes

Critics of the SOAP format state that the information focuses on the patient's impairments, implying that improvement in these will improve the patient's functional abilities. When Dr. Lawrence Weed introduced the POMR and the SOAP note, documentation content, in the 1960's, he did focus on the impairments (see Chapters 1, 2). Although a SOAP-organized note can be written about functional outcomes, as seen in the earlier crutch-training example, a variety of other formats can be designed with a clearer focus on functional outcomes.

Information in the medical record is recorded in a variety of formats. Notes are written as a narrative paragraph or as a SOAP outline. Flow charts, graphs, checklists, and fill-in-the-blank forms are often used in hospitals and rehabilitation centers, whereas private practice therapists may put the information into a letter to the physician. In schools, the child's treatment plan and goals are incorporated into an IEP. Medicare information is documented on standardized Medicare forms. (Refer to Chapter 2 for examples.) In addition, other disciplines responsible for the patient's care may also provide subjective data (refer to Box 2–3).

Relevant Information

One of the key words in the definition for subjective data is *relevant*. Unfortunately, a common mistake seen in progress notes is the inclusion of information that does not relate to the patient's problem, diagnosis, or the treatment session (Fig. 3–2). Confining the subjective information to only that which is relevant is not an easy task. The PTA and the patient will likely have conversations about a variety of subjects. Important information about the patient's problem or diagnosis often slips out during a seemingly unrelated conversation. The PTA must be an alert listener to sort out the relevant information.

Necessary Listening Skills

Effective listening is a skill that is consciously developed with practice. To sort out relevant information, the PTA must be aware that much of the workday is spent listening in a variety of ways. Listening techniques include:

1. **Analytic** listening for specific kinds of information (e.g., pain, lifestyle, fears)
2. **Directed** listening to a patient's answers to specific questions (e.g., What positions increase frequency or intensity of pain? What does the patient need to be able to do their work?)
3. **Attentive** listening for general information to get the total picture of the patient's situation (e.g., What are the physical barriers at the patient's home or place of employment?)
4. **Exploratory** listening because of one's own interest in the subject
5. **Appreciative** listening for aesthetic pleasure (e.g., listening to music on headphones while walking during lunch break)
6. **Courteous** listening because it demonstrates respect for the patient
7. **Passive** listening by overhearing (e.g., conversation in the next treatment booth)

11-17-06   **Dx:** Ⓛ CVA.
   PT Dx: Weakness in Ⓡ UE & LE with unsafe ambulation and dependent in ADLs.
   Pt. states not doing exercises at home; has not been going out to church or club meetings because she is afraid of falling. Pt. states she has always been active and wishes she could go to her bridge club meetings. She loves to play bridge and misses her bridge club friends the most. They have been friends since they were girls together in grade school. They just celebrated their 65th year of friendship!

   Robert Relevant, SPTA/ Tom Jones, PTA

Figure 3—2   Subjective data section of a progress note containing superfluous information.

4-19-06 PT Dx: Subdeltoid bursitis with decreased deltoid strength and decreased shoulder ROM interfering with ability to perform work tasks.

S: Pt. reports itching "right where the PT gave my first ultrasound treatment yesterday." Mentioned she is allergic to some perfumes.

O: No skin rash or redness observable in treatment area today. Direct contact US/1 MHz/1.5 w/cm² (moderate heat)/5 min/(R) subdeltoid bursa/sitting/shoulder extended/arm resting on pillow to decrease inflammation. Used ultrasound lotion instead of gel. Gel contains perfume. Pt. correctly performed home exercise program of isometrics for the deltoid, holding for 8 counts (see copy in chart).

Shoulder

AROM:	before tx	after tx
flexion	0–55°	0–60°
abduction	0–68°	0–73°

A: Treatment tissue less sensitive to US (1 w/cm² yesterday). US effective in reducing inflammation. Pt. beginning to progress toward goal of decreased inflammation, improved shoulder mobility to perform work tasks.

P: Will monitor pt.'s response to the US lotion tomorrow and alert PT of the reaction to the gel. Pt. is scheduled for four more treatments.—Sue Citizen, PTA

Figure 3–3 Adding new relevant subjective information to the medical record through the progress note.

Analytic, directed, and attentive listening provide information that may be relevant as subjective data in the progress note. (Fig. 3–3) More relevant information may be revealed when exploratory listening is used.

ORGANIZING SUBJECTIVE DATA

The subjective content in the initial examination report may be more complex and detailed than the subjective information in the progress note. The PT may organize this information into subcategories, such as complaints (c/o), history (Hx), environment, the patient's goals or functional outcomes, behavior, and pain. This helps the PT confine the data to only those categories that are relevant. Organizing the content makes it easy to read and to locate information. The example in Figure 3–4 randomly presents subjective data, making it difficult to get a clear picture of the patient's status. In Figure 3–5, the note is rewritten with the information grouped according to topic.

The PTA needs to document subjective data only if there is an update of the previous information or if there is relevant new information. Usually the content is brief. If the information is about more than one topic category, it should be grouped according to the topics. However, identifying the topic categories may not be necessary. Progress notes may not contain subjective information when relevant information is not provided or when the patient is unable to communicate (e.g., the patient is in a coma) and there is no one else present during the treatment to offer subjective data.

WRITING SUBJECTIVE DATA

Verbs

When documenting subjective data, use verbs to indicate to the reader that the information is being provided by the patient. Commonly used verbs include *states, reports, complains of, expresses, describes,* and *denies.* It is not necessary to repeat the word *patient* (or pt.) After it is used once, it is assumed that all the information in the section was told by the patient, as in the examples in Figure 3–6.

Patient Quotations

Occasionally, using direct patient quotations is better than paraphrasing the patient's comments. Quoting will make the intent of the comment or the relevance to the treatment clearer. The following are appropriate situations in which to quote the patient:

Pt. c/o pain in (R) shoulder when (R) arm is hanging down. Lives alone. Pt.'s goal is to play on the college volleyball team this winter. Denies having previous injury or trauma to shoulder. C/o pain when attempting to put on sweater and T-shirts. States he is limited to only a few clothing items he can get into without help. States his shoulder started to ache for no apparent reason. Has been practicing volleyball 6 hr/day for the last 3 weeks.

Figure 3–4 Documentation that randomly presents subjective data, making it difficult to get a clear picture of patient's status.

> **c/o:** Pt. c/o pain Ⓡ shoulder when Ⓡ arm is hanging down and when attempting to put on sweater and T-shirts. **Hx:** States his shoulder started to ache for no apparent reason. Denies having previous injury or trauma to shoulder. **Home situation:** States lives alone. Has only a few clothing items he can get into without help. **Environment/pt.'s goals:** States he has been practicing volleyball 6 hr/day for the last 3 weeks. Wants to play on the college volleyball team this winter.

Figure 3—5   The information in Figure 3-4 rewritten with the information grouped according to topics.

> 1) Patient states she's allergic to perfume; itched at treatment site following yesterday's treatment. 2) Patient states he is anxious to go fishing; has six steps down to the dock at his cabin. 3) Patient reports he awoke only three times last night; denies having leg tingling and back soreness.

Figure 3—6   Three examples of documentation using the word *patient* once.

1. To illustrate confusion or loss of memory. (*Example:* Pt. often states, "My mother is coming to take me away from here. I want my mother." Pt. is 90 years old.)
2. To illustrate denial. (*Example:* Pt. insists, "I don't need any help at home. I'll be fine once I get home." Pt. is dependent for transfers and ambulation and lives alone.)
3. To illustrate a patient's attitude toward therapy. (*Example:* Pt. states, "I don't want to play children's games. If I could just go home, I would be fine.")
4. To illustrate the patient's use of abusive language. (*Example:* Pt. yelled to therapist, "Keep your hands off my arm! I'm going to kill you!")

Information From Someone Other Than the Patient   Relevant information is often provided by the caretaker or significant other. This is especially true for patients with dementia, speech dysfunction, and altered neurologic function, such as coma, and for infants and young children.

When the information is provided by someone other than the patient, begin the subjective information by stating who provided the information. Be sure to state the reason why the patient could not communicate. (*Example:* All of the following information is provided by pt.'s mother. Pt. is in a coma.) When information is provided by both the patient and another person, specifically note when it is patient-supplied information and when the information is supplied by the other person. (*Example:* Mrs. Jones states she did not have to help her husband button his sweater today. Mr. Jones states that today is the first time he has not had to ask for help since his arthritis flared up.)

Pain   Documentation of pain is unique because it often seems like objective data (Fig. 3–7). Also, it may seem as though pain is the judgment or opinion of the therapist. Pain is an element of the subjective data content. Pain information is placed in the S (subjective) section of the SOAP-organized progress note.

A patient's pain experience and perception of its intensity vary widely among individuals. Consider the example of dental experiences; some dental patients never need local anesthesia to have a cavity filled, whereas others need Novocain (procaine hydrochloride), music in headphones, and other distractions.

> 1. Patient rates pain a 6 on an ascending scale of 1–10 when climbing stairs.
> 2. Patient gives her pain a 4 on a pain scale of 1–7 where 1 is no pain and 7 is excruciating pain.
> 3. Patient reports his pain is 3/10 after massage compared to 6/10 before massage.
> 4. 1_____x_____1
>   1 2 3 4 5 6 7 8 9 10

Figure 3—7   How the documentation of pain looks like objective data.

Pain is difficult to describe in words. Not only can patients experiencing similar levels of pain use different words to describe that pain, but different therapists may attribute different meaning to patients' words. Because the patient is providing the pain description, this information is documented in the subjective section.

Each facility has its own procedure for documenting pain. Typically, this information is documented in the pain profile. Several types of pain profiles are commonly used, including pain scales, checklists, and body drawings. Regardless of the pain profile or technique used for documenting the pain, consistency in each note is essential. Inconsistent documentation hinders a determination of treatment effectiveness. Information on a pain scale cannot be compared with information on a body drawing. Changes in the pain profile can be identified by comparing the initial profile with the pain reports throughout the treatment sessions.

Consistent pain documentation provides a clear picture or measurement of treatment effectiveness and helps ensure reimbursement by third-party payers. It is important to understand that, although the pain profile provides an *objective* method for documenting pain, pain is documented in the *subjective* section of the progress note. Students often make the mistake of documenting pain in the objective section.

Pain Scale   Facilities often use a pain profile based on a numbered scale, usually from 0 to 10 or 1 to 7 with 0 or 1 denoting no pain and 7 or 10 denoting the worst pain imaginable. The patient rates the pain as a number on the scale. This information is recorded in the subjective section (see Fig. 3–7). The scale should be described in the note (e.g., "0" = no pain, "10" = worst pain imaginable; "1" is no pain, "7" is excruciating," "on an ascending scale of 0–10.") The pain rating may be documented as 5/10 or 3/7 if the definition of the scale has been described earlier in the record or chart.

Checklist   Another method of documenting pain is a checklist of words describing pain. The patient checks the words that describe his pain. This checklist is inserted in the medical chart, and a note in the subjective section of the progress note instructs the reader to refer to the checklist. Figure 3–8 is an example of a checklist pain profile.

There are many words that describe pain. Some of these are grouped below. Check (✓) any words that describe the pain you have these days.

1.	5.	9.	13.	17.
☐ Flickering	☐ Pinching	☐ Dull	☐ Fearful	☐ Spreading
☐ Quivering	☐ Pressing	☐ Sore	☐ Frightful	☐ Radiating
☐ Pulsing	☐ Gnawing	☐ Hurting	☐ Terrifying	☐ Penetrating
☐ Throbbing	☐ Cramping	☐ Aching		☐ Piercing
☐ Beating	☐ Crushing	☐ Heavy		
☐ Pounding				

2.	6.	10.	14.	18.
☐ Jumping	☐ Tugging	☐ Tender	☐ Punishing	☐ Tight
☐ Flashing	☐ Pulling	☐ Taut	☐ Grueling	☐ Numb
☐ Shooting	☐ Wrenching	☐ Rasping	☐ Cruel	☐ Drawing
		☐ Splitting	☐ Vicious	☐ Squeezing
			☐ Killing	☐ Tearing

3.	7.	11.	15.	19.
☐ Pricking	☐ Hot	☐ Tiring	☐ Wretched	☐ Cool
☐ Boring	☐ Burning	☐ Exhausting	☐ Blinding	☐ Cold
☐ Drilling	☐ Scalding			☐ Freezing
☐ Stabbing	☐ Searing			

4.	8.	12.	16.	20.
☐ Sharp	☐ Tingling	☐ Sickening	☐ Annoying	☐ Nagging
☐ Cutting	☐ Itchy	☐ Suffocating	☐ Troublesome	☐ Nauseating
☐ Lacerating	☐ Smarting		☐ Miserable	☐ Agonizing
	☐ Stinging		☐ Intense	☐ Dreadful
			☐ Unbearable	☐ Torturing

Figure 3–8   An example of a checklist pain profile (Adapted from the McGill Pain Questionnaire).

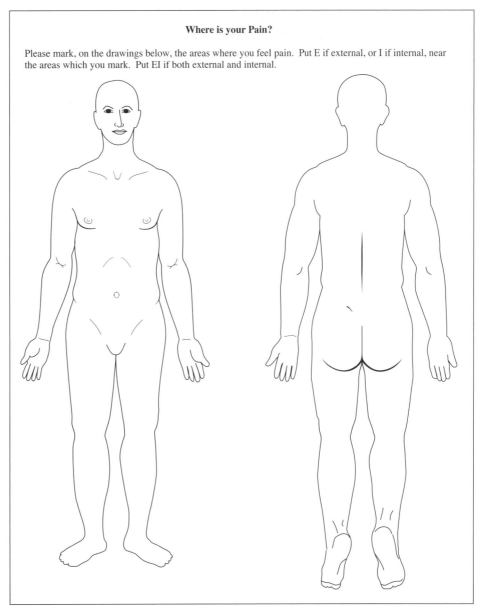

Where is your Pain?

Please mark, on the drawings below, the areas where you feel pain. Put E if external, or I if internal, near the areas which you mark. Put EI if both external and internal.

Figure 3—9   An example of a body-drawing pain profile.

Body Drawing   An outline drawing of the body may be used by the patient to mark the location of the pain. Symbols or colors are used to indicate the type and intensity of the pain at each location. This form is then inserted in the medical chart for pain documentation. Figure 3–9 is an example of a body drawing pain profile.

SUMMARY   Information told to the PT or PTA by the patient, significant other, or other caregiver is documented as subjective data in the progress note. The information must be relevant to the patient's physical therapy diagnosis or treatment. The PT and PTA use different types of listening to identify relevant information. This information can be paraphrased or quoted verbatim in the progress note. Including subjective information in the progress note when none was provided or when the patient repeated information that has already been documented in previous notes is not necessary. Although appearing more like objective data, comments regarding pain and structured pain profiles are documented with the subjective data.

REFERENCES   1. *Person-first language.* Accessed on March 15, 2007 from http://www.asha.org/about/publications/journals-abstracts/submissions/person_first.
2. American Physical Therapy Association. (June 2003). *The guide to physical therapist practice.* APTA, Alexandria, VA.

Review Exercises

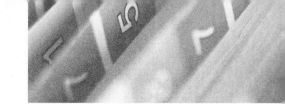

1. Describe the information documented in the **subjective** section of a SOAP note.

2. Explain the **responsibilities** for documentation for the PT and the PTA.

3. What is **subjective** data?

4. List **two** examples of appropriate and inappropriate subjective statements.

5. What should the PTA do if he or she finds an **inappropriate** subjective statement in the patient chart?

6. Why is **subjective information** important in patient documentation?

7. Documentation procedures are different in each physical therapy clinic. What **rule** should the PTA follow?

PRACTICE EXERCISES

Practice Exercise 1 ➤ *Think of two events that occurred recently in your life (e.g., car problem and how you solved it, lost keys and how they were found), and write about them in SOAP format. Organize the information so what is told to you (subjective data) is in the S section, measurable happenings and things you observed (objective data) are in the O section, the meaning of or your conclusions about the data (assessment) are in the A section, and what you plan to do next is in the P section. Write one of your notes in outline form with SOAP headings, as shown in the notes on pages 52 and 56. Write one of the notes in paragraph form with the information sequenced in SOAP organization but without headings.*

S_____

O_____

A_____

P_____

_____

_____

_____

_____

Practice Exercise 2 ➤ *You have treated your patient and have taken notes about the treatment session. Identify the "S" sections of the SOAP note.*

_____ Outcome ① sit to stand met.

_____ Observed patient sitting in middle of couch.

_____ Patient expresses frustration can't get up from couch without help, especially in evening.

_____ Dx: Multiple sclerosis.

_____ Gross MMT 32/5 all LE muscle groups, 2/5 initial eval.

_____ PT Dx: LE weakness limiting ability to sit ↔ stand and ambulate safely.

_____ Patient sat at end of couch, scooted forward to edge, used couch arm to help push up. 3rd trial able to sit to stand ①, verbal cues to lean forward.

_____ Instructed patient not to sit on couch in evening when fatigued and weaker.

_____ Strength gain LEs.

_____ Will visit patient 2 more times and schedule PT's discharge evaluation.

Practice Exercise 3 ➤ *Rewrite this unorganized note so the subjective information is located at the beginning of the note.*

3-26-06:

_____

Pt. has met his short-term outcome of ① crutch walking on level and uneven ground. Says he needs to be able to climb three flights of stairs to get to his apartment. Will work on stair climbing next session. Handrail on Ⓛ going up. Pt. ambulated, NWB Ⓡ, axillary crutches, Ⓘ on grass and uneven sidewalk, 300 ft Ⓡ ankle & foot edema. Circumference equals Ⓛ foot & ankle measurements (see initial eval). All Ⓡ ankle AROM WNL, Ⓡ knee flexion PROM 10°–110° (15°–100° last session). Pt. correctly demonstrated self-knee ROM & gentle stretching exercises (see copy in chart). RLE mobility progressing. Will inform PT that pt. will be ready for discharge evaluation next session. Limited RLE mobility and NWB because of Fx Ⓡ femur, pinned 3-22-06.

—Confused Student, SPTA/Puzzled Therapist, PT (Lic. #420)

_____

_____

_____

_____

Practice Exercise 4 ➤ *Identify the subjective information from the following list of statements by placing an "S" in the space provided.*

_____ Sam Smart, PTA (Lic. #007)

_____ Patient c/o itching around wound.

_____ 6/10/00

_____ Wound healing as diameter is 2 cm smaller than at initial treatment.

_____ During gait training, pt. Ⓘ ambulated with axillary crutches, toe-touch gait pattern for left, on grass, curbs, sidewalk, carpeting, in/out car, stairs.

_____ Good posture, good step-through gait.

_____ Whirlpool/105°F/sitting/Ⓛ heel/to remove dressings/10 min

_____ Outcome for independent ambulation in home and community met.

_____ Will report to PT re: d/c gait training.

_____ Will continue wound care per POC.

_____ Diameter wound 4 cm (6 cm initial treatment).

_____ Teaspoon drainage, clear, no odor.

_____ Wound pink.

_____ Goal for healed wound 50% met.

_____ Patient says feels comfortable and safe on crutches.

_____ Sterile dressings applied per previous treatment procedures.

Practice Exercise 5 ➤   *You have been treating your patient who had a* Ⓡ *CVA with* Ⓛ *hemiplegia, following the treatment plan on the cardex (see Fig. 2–9). Your patient has progressed, and the cardex needs to be updated, especially because you will be on vacation next week and another PTA will be seeing your patient. The patient reports that her pain level has decreased from a 9/10 during the last session to a 6/10 today. The changes include the following: 5 reps active assistive* Ⓛ *scapular protraction in supine with active assistive elbow extension facilitated by tapping triceps muscle belly, RUE PREs 2 lb, 10×/3 lb, 10×/4 lb as many reps as can (stop at 10), 5-lb cuff wts., for all RLE exercises, ambulation in // bars 2× with max. assist of 2 to facilitate wt. shift to* Ⓛ *and control knee, using temporary AFO on* Ⓛ *ankle, sitting sitting balance now min. assist of 1, now* Ⓘ *with w/c mobility as brings self to therapy. Standing table discontinued. Other* Ⓛ *UE exercises the same.*

1. Document these findings on the following form:

DX: _____   INITIAL DATE: _____

PRECAUTIONS: _____   UPDATE: _____

Exercise	set	rep	equipment	assist	Goals
					TDD:
					TDP:

Patient Name	Age	Sex	MD	PT	RM#	Units

Transfers	Method	Assist	Other

Pregait/Gait

2. Identify the **subjective** information in the note above.

_____

_____

_____

_____

Practice Exercise 6 ➤ *Place a check mark next to the sentences that would go in the subjective section of documentation of patient care.*

_____ The patient stated that she likes the PTA's new shoes.

_____ The patient's husband confirmed that the patient took her pain medication a half hour before her physical therapy appointment.

_____ The PT stated that the patient will continue working on the current home exercise program until the patient can ambulate independently.

_____ Patient demonstrated normal range of motion in the Ⓡ elbow.

_____ The patient stated that she has a job interview tomorrow and will not be able to attend her therapy appointment.

_____ The patient was able to ambulate independently on uneven surfaces up to 30 ft with axillary crutches.

_____ The patient's wife said that they are going shopping at the new bookstore after he is done with his therapy.

_____ Patient will be seen once a week for physical therapy at the outpatient clinic.

_____ The patient became fatigued after walking 20 ft with the FWW.

_____ The patient said that she is motivated to do well in her physical therapy so she can return to her hobby of roller derby.

Practice Exercise 7 ➤ *Make corrections to the "S" section of the following SOAP note. Some sentences may need to be omitted.*

S: He was seen today for a physical therapy session in his home as per the PT's plan of care. She said that he woke up frequently last night complaining of pain in his lower back. The patient was able to sit in a chair for 15 min while doing his exercises. He rated his pain at a 7/10 while performing his exercises. His daughter said that the patient completed all of his exercises twice yesterday afternoon.

_____

_____

_____

_____

_____

_____

Practice Exercise 8 ➤ *Write "Pr" next to statements that describe the physical therapy problem or diagnosis and "S" next to statements that fit the subjective data category.*

_____ Pt. states she has a clear understanding of her disease and her prognosis.

_____ Pt. expresses surprise that the ice massage relaxed her muscle spasm.

_____ Muscle spasms Ⓛ lumbar paraspinals with sitting tolerance limited to 10 min.

_____ Pt. describes tingling pain down back of Ⓡ leg to heel.

_____ Dependent in ADLs because of flaccid paralysis in Ⓡ upper and lower extremities.

_____ Sue states her Ⓛ ear hurts.

_____ Unable to reach behind back because of limited ROM in Ⓡ shoulder int. rot.

_____ Reports he must be able to return to work as a welder.

_____ Patient states the doctor told her she had a laceration in her Ⓡ vastus medialis.

_____ Paraplegic 2° SCI T12 and dependent in wheelchair transfers.

_____ States Hx of RA since 1980.

_____ Pt. denies pain c̄ cough.

_____ States injury occurred December 31, 1999.

_____ SPTA c/o he has to sit for 2 hours in the PTA lectures.

_____ Grip strength weakness and inability to turn doorknobs because of carpal tunnel syndrome.

_____ Describes his pain as "burning."

_____ Unable to sit because of decubitus over sacrum.

_____ Unable to feed self because of limited elbow flexion.

_____ Pt. rates her pain a 4 on an ascending scale of 1–10.

_____ States able to sit through a 2-hour movie last night.

Practice Exercise 9 ➤ *Follow the directions in the next three questions.*

1. For each of the statements in Practice Exercise 8 to which you answered "Pr," *underline* the impairment and *circle* the functional limitation.

2. For each of the statements in Practice Exercise 8 to which you answered "S," *underline* the verb in the statement that specified it was subjective.

3. List the medical diagnoses you can find in the statements.

_____

_____

_____

_____

_____

_____

Practice Exercise 10 ➤ *Place "Yes" next to relevant subjective data statements and "No" next to those that do not seem relevant.*

_____ 1. Client stated her dog was hit by a car last night and she felt too depressed today to do her exercises.

_____ 2. Client reported he progressed his exercises to 50 push-ups yesterday.

_____ 3. Patient's daughter stated she traveled from Iowa, where it has been raining for 2 weeks.

_____ 4. Patient states he does not like the hospital food and is hungry for some Dairy Queen.

_____ 5. Patient rates her pain a 4 on an ascending scale of 1–7.

_____ 6. Patient states she is now able to reach the second shelf of her kitchen cupboard to reach for a glass.

_____ 7. Patient reports he had this same tingling discomfort in his right foot 3 years ago.

_____ 8. Client reports experiencing an aching in his "elbow bone" after the ultrasound treatment yesterday.

_____ 9. Patient says she has 10 grandchildren and 4 great grandchildren.

_____ 10. Client states she forgot to tell the PT that she loves to bowl.

_____ 11. Client reports that *ER* is his favorite TV program.

_____ 12. Client reports he sat in his fishing boat 3 hours and caught a 7-pound Northern Pike this weekend.

_____ 13. Client states he played golf yesterday for the first time since his back injury.

_____ 14. Client states he shot a 56 in golf.

_____ 15. Client states she cannot turn her head to look over her shoulder to back the car out of the garage.

_____ 16. Patient's mother wants to know when her son will come out of the coma.

_____ 17. Client reports he wishes he had not been drinking beer the night of his accident.

_____ 18. Patient describes his flight of stairs with 10 steps, a landing, then 5 more steps and the railing on the right when going up.

_____ 19. Client wishes it would rain, as her prize roses are dying.

_____ 20. Patient states, "I'm going to Macy's to shop and have lunch today." (Patient is 89 years old and is a resident in a long-term-care facility in a small town in Ohio. She has been placed on some new medication.)

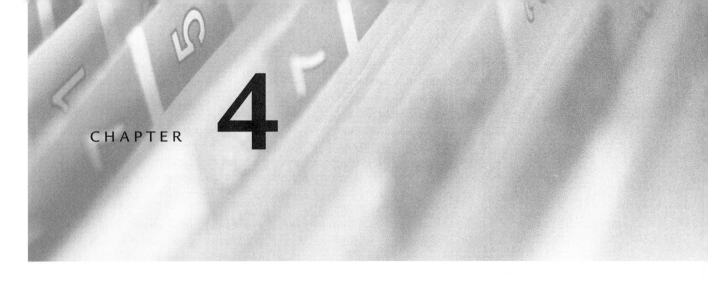

CHAPTER **4**

What Is Objective Data and Why It Is Important

LEARNING OBJECTIVES　*After studying this chapter, the student will be able to:*

- ☐ Identify objective data.
- ☐ Organize objective data for easy reading and understanding.
- ☐ Demonstrate adherence to recommended guidelines for documenting objective data.
- ☐ Document the patient's functional abilities to provide the reader with a picture of patient functioning.
- ☐ Document interventions so they are reproducible by another PTA or a PT.
- ☐ Document objective data consistent with the data in the PT's initial examination.
- ☐ Identify common mistakes students typically make when documenting objective data.
- ☐ Explain the difference between subjective and objective information.

INTRODUCTION　The *"O,"* or *objective, section* contains the objective data; that is, data that can be reproduced or confirmed by another professional with the same training as the person gathering the objective information. This information is gathered by measurable and reproducible tests and observations. It must be described in terms of functional movement or actions. These are the **signs** of the patient's disease or dysfunction and are recorded in the objective section. This section is a summary, "painting a picture" about the patient.

　　　The objective data in the PT's examination report and the PTA's progress note are included with or immediately after the subjective data. These data make up the content of the O (objective) section of the SOAP outline, are included in the data section of the DEP note, are part of the status information in the PSPG-organized note, and are the physical therapy assessment information in the FOR.

The reader of the objective data in the PTA's progress note should be able to form a mental picture of the patient, the interventions performed, the patient's response to the interventions, and the patient's functioning before and after the interventions. The PTA should write the objective data so the words paint a picture of the patient and the treatment session. The reader should also be able to clearly understand that the interventions provided during the treatment session require the skills of a trained physical therapy provider (PT or PTA).

OBJECTIVE DATA

Objective data include any information that can be reproduced or observed by someone else with the same training (i.e., another PT or PTA). When written, objective data provide the reader not trained in physical therapy with an understanding of the treatment session and with sufficient information to determine whether or not the patient is benefiting from physical therapy. The PTA writes the objective section with two audiences in mind: (1) another PTA (e.g., a replacement PTA in the event you are unable to report to work); and (2) a reader untrained in physical therapy (e.g., an insurance representative, lawyer, quality assurance committee member, physician, or other health-care provider) who is determining the effectiveness of the treatment session.

ORGANIZING OBJECTIVE DATA

Five general topics are appropriate for objective data in the progress note:

1. The results of measurements and tests
2. A description of the patient's function
3. A description of the interventions provided
4. The PTA's objective observations of the patient
5. A record of the number of treatment sessions provided

The information in the objective section of the progress note is organized to flow from one topic to the next, thus making the information easy to read. Similar information should be grouped together. For example, intervention descriptions, results of measurements and tests, and descriptions of the patient's functioning should be organized into three distinct groups.

WRITING OBJECTIVE DATA

The objective data about the initial examination consist of information relevant to the patient's chief complaint and the reason the patient is seeking physical therapy care. These data form the basis for designing the treatment outcomes, goals, and plan. The objective data must consist of measurable, reproducible information so the efficacy of physical therapy treatment procedures can be determined through research of the progress note. When appropriate, the PTA should relate the objective data in the progress note to the same information in the initial examination report or in previous notes for comparison. Some objective data can be charted or graphed to provide a quick picture of progress.

Results of Measurements and Tests

All the activities or areas specifically mentioned in the initial examination reporting the outcomes and goals in the evaluation report should be reassessed and recorded in the progress notes and in the interim and discharge evaluation reports. The PTA determines the patient's progress by readministering the measurements and tests performed in the initial examination that the PTA is trained to perform. These results are then compared with the results either in the initial examination report or in previous progress notes, if the patient has been receiving physical therapy for a long period of time. For the comparison to be valid, the retest or measurement must follow the same procedures and techniques that were used when the initial examination was performed. The documentation of the results must also be consistent. For example, if the measurements were in centimeters in the initial examination, they should continue to be documented in centimeters.

The documentation of results may be in the form of either a comment referring the reader to previous results (e.g., "See distance walked in note dated 8-2-06") or an actual written comparison with the results of the previous measurements or tests. Consider the following example.

Center Ⓛ lat. malleolus	**8-10-00**	**8-15-00**
1" inferior to center Ⓛ lat. malleolus	6"	4"
1" superior to center Ⓛ lat. malleolus	5.5"	3"
All measurements taken along the superior edge of the marks.	6"	4"

Figure 4–1   Documentation of measurements in a table form.

Example: PTA Sam is treating Mr. Wilson with compression pump therapy to decrease edema in the Ⓛ ankle. Measurements of the circumference of Mr. Wilson's Ⓛ ankle were taken in the initial examination (on 8-10-06) to determine the extent of the edema. Today, after 5 treatments, Sam remeasures the circumference of the ankle and compares his results with the initial examination measurements to prove that the edema has decreased and the compression pump intervention is effective. Sam could record the measurements in a table format in the objective section for easy comparison. Figure 4–1 illustrates measurements presented in table form.

In this example, the reader can easily compare results and see that the edema has decreased and the patient is benefiting from the compression pump intervention. Another PTA could follow the directions and duplicate the measurement procedure. Other measurements and tests performed by PTAs, with guidelines for documenting the results, are described in Box 4–1.

Description of the Patient's Function

The PTA documents improvement by describing the patient's function. For example, at the initial examination, Mr. Wilson could not fit his Ⓛ foot into his running shoe because of the edema in the Ⓛ foot and ankle. Today, he was able to get his Ⓛ foot into the shoe with the help of a shoehorn. The next day, another PTA could duplicate the assessment by watching Mr. Wilson use a shoehorn to put on his left running shoe. This is a good way to document intervention effectiveness because it paints a picture of the patient and describes clearly how the physical therapy interventions are improving the patient's ability to function in his environment. The functional activities must be those specifically mentioned in the goals or functional outcomes in the initial evaluation.

When a comparison of the data shows that the patient's functional status has not changed, be sure all methods for measuring change have been used. For example, a patient may continue to need the assistance of one person for ambulation, but the time it takes the patient to walk from the bed to the bathroom has decreased. Include the following information when describing the patient's function:

- The function (e.g., ambulation, transferring, stair climbing, lifting, sweeping, sitting, standing, moving from sit to stand or stand to sit)
- Quality of the movement when performing the function (e.g., even weight-bearing, smooth movement, correct body mechanics, speed)
- Level of assistance needed (i.e., ranging from independence; verbal reminders; tactile guidance; supervision; standby assist or contact guard assist; minimal, moderate, maximal assist; to dependent)
- Purpose of the assistance (e.g., verbal cueing for gait pattern, for recovery of loss of balance, for added strength, to monitor weight-bearing, to guide walker)
- Equipment needed (e.g., ambulation aids, orthotics, supports, railings, wheelchair, assistive devices)
- Distances, heights, lengths, times, weights (e.g., 300 feet, 10 meters, 6 minutes, top shelf of standard-height kitchen cabinet, floor to table, 20 pounds)
- Environmental conditions (e.g., level surface, carpeting, dim light, outside, ramps, low seat)
- Cognitive status and any complicating factors (patient understanding, ability to follow directions, fainting easily, blood pressure needing monitoring)

Box 4–1   Other Measurements and Tests Performed By PTAs with Guidelines for Documenting the Results

Guidelines

All measurements and tests must be performed and documented in the same manner as they were performed and documented in the PT initial evaluation. The documentation should include, when applicable:

1. Exactly what is being measured or tested, and on which side.
2. If a motion is being tested, is it active or passive?
3. The position of the patient.
4. The starting and ending points, the boundaries, and the measurement points above and below the starting point.
5. The same scale (e.g., inches, centimeters, degrees) that was used in the initial evaluation.

Measurements
· Tape Measurements
· Girth or circumference
· Leg length
· Wound size
· Step and stride length
· Neck and trunk range of motion
· Goniometry of all joints

Tests
· Manual muscle test of muscle groups
· Gross sensory testing

Vital Signs
· Heart rate
· Respiratory rate
· Blood pressure

Standardized Functional Tests*
· Functional Independence Measure
· Barthel Assessment
· Tinetti Balance
· Peabody Developmental Motor Scales
· Duke Mobility Status
· Posture

---

*These are examples of the many tests available.

Standardized Functional Assessments

For assessing functional abilities, many tools with set protocols and procedures, clear instructions, and methods for rating or scoring the level of function are available. A few examples of these tests are the Tinetti Balance Test, Peabody Developmental Motor Scales, Barthel Assessment, Duke Mobility Skills, and Functional Independence Measure. If a standardized assessment tool is used in the initial examination, the PTA, when trained in the use of the tool, can reassess the patient's functional abilities and refer the reader of the progress note to the copy of the completed assessment form in the chart. The assessment tool describes the function and changes in the rating score as evidence of improvement in functional abilities and progress toward the functional outcome identified in the initial evaluation.

Description of the Interventions Provided

The objective data may include information about the treatment parameters, sets and repetitions of exercises, or other tests and measurements that can be recorded. The interventions may be described in the progress note, recorded on a flow chart, or described on a separate form elsewhere in the medical record. In addition, this information may be a combination of narrative progress notes with a checklist type chart. Besides being recorded in the medical record, the interventions are often detailed on a cardex located in the physical therapy department. The PTA should follow the procedures of the facility.

Intervention details must be complete and thorough so the intervention can be duplicated by another PT or PTA. The following information should be included for the intervention description to be reproducible.

1. Identification of the modality, exercise, or activity
2. Dosage, number of repetitions, and distance
3. Identification of the exact piece of equipment, when applicable
4. Settings of dials or programs on equipment
5. Target tissue or treatment area
6. Purpose of the treatment
7. Patient positioning
8. Duration, frequency, and rest breaks
9. Other information that the therapist needs to be aware of that is outside standard procedure or protocol. For example, a cane is adjusted higher than the height determined by standard procedure because the increased height provided greater assistance to the patient for ambulation.
10. Anything that is unique to the treatment of that particular patient; for example, complicating factors, such as taking the patient's pulse rate every 5 minutes.

Appendix B provides guidelines for documenting specific direct interventions.

The intervention description should include or be combined with a description of the patient's response to the intervention. For example: Decreased muscle spasm (decreased muscle tone) was palpable following ice massage, due to numbing response (7 min), Ⓛ paraspinal mms, L3–5, with pt. prone over one pillow.

The details of the intervention can also be included to describe function. For example: Following instructions, pt. safely ambulated with axillary crutches, no wt.-bearing on Ⓛ, from bed to dining room (50 ft) on tiled level surface with standby assist for support for loss of balance recovery 2X.

In these two examples, a reader untrained in physical therapy can visualize the patient's performance, and another PTA could duplicate the interventions the following day.

A copy of any written instructions or information provided to the patient as part of the treatment session should be placed in the medical record. Frequently, the PTA will give the patient or a caregiver written instructions for exercises or activities that were taught during the treatment session. This is noted in the objective data, and the reader is informed that a copy is in the chart. When the reader can reproduce the intervention by following the written instructions on the handout, it is not necessary to describe the exercises in the progress note. Figure 4–2 illustrates objective documentation of a treatment session that includes instructing the patient in a home exercise program. In the objective data section, any equipment that was given, lent, or sold to the patient should be mentioned.

PTA's Objective Patient Observations A description of what the PTA sees or feels (visual and tactile observations) constitutes objective data if it is an observation that another PT or PTA would also make because they have the same training. The observation could be duplicated or confirmed by another PT or PTA. Two examples of objective observations are (1) reddened skin over a bony area after applica-

---

O: Following verbal instructions and demonstrations, pt. accurately performed home exercise program designed to strengthen Ⓡ hip abductors, extensors, and quadriceps, 5 reps of each ex. today. Pt. provided written instructions, refer to copy in chart.

O: Pt. accurately demonstrated set-up of home cervical polyaxial traction unit; gave self 10-min intermittent traction,15 lb, approximately 5 sec on, 3 sec off, supine. Pt. provided written instructions, see copy in chart.

Figure 4–2 Objective documentation of a treatment session that included instructing the patient in a home exercise program.

tion of hot packs, such as "a nickel-size, reddened area noted over inferior angle of left scapular after hot pack treatment," and (2) a description of the patient's gait pattern or how the patient walks, such as "client walks with an antalgic gait; trunk held in a slightly forward-leaning posture, minimal arm swing, no pelvic rotation, uneven step length (shorter on right), and shortened stance time on right."

Proof of the Necessity for Skilled Physical Therapy Services

The reader of the progress note must come to the conclusion that the physical therapy services the patient received required the unique skills of physical therapy-trained personnel. With this in mind, the PTA should constantly be mentally asking, "Could someone not trained in physical therapy do what I have just described?" If the instructions presented in this chapter are being followed, the PTA is well on the way to writing the objective data so it describes the need for skilled services. Comparing the objective data in the progress note with the objective data in the initial examination is one way of proving that skilled services are needed.

Careful selection of words also is important. For example, PTs and PTAs do not walk/ambulate or transfer their patients; they *teach* or *train* their patients to ambulate or transfer. Therefore, the intervention described in the progress note should be listed as *gait training* or *transfer training.* The note should describe the patient's response to the training or indicate whether the patient understood the instructions or learned the skill or technique (e.g., "During gait training, patient ambulated with axillary crutches, NWB on left, needing contact guard assist for security when recovering from occasional loss of balance, 30 ft on carpeting, 5X, responding to verbal cues for correct posture and proper step-through pattern but needing frequent cueing first 2X and improving to needing one cue by 5X"). When the patient is taught something, such as exercises, body mechanics, or posture, the note should document that the patient gave a return demonstration of what was taught and whether the demonstration was correct or the patient needed further instructions. Again, the note should use words to "paint a picture" of the patient.

Record of Treatment Sessions

The progress note should keep track of the patient's attendance by recording the number of treatment sessions that have been provided. "Documenting attendance reflects the patient's compliance and participation in rehabilitation."[1] The note should also identify appointments that the patient did not keep and the reason for not attending. When a third-party payer has limited the number of treatment sessions that a patient may receive, the progress note can be a method for tracking the number of sessions for discharge planning. The objective data section can report the number of times the patient has been treated, and the information in the plan section of the note can state how many more treatment sessions are scheduled in the future.

Common Student Mistakes With Objective Data Documentation

The major mistake PTA students make when writing objective data, especially when documenting the interventions provided, is reporting what they did and not how the patient responded or performed; for example, "Instructed pt. in crutch walking, non–wt.-bearing Ⓛ."

This statement refers to what the therapist did. However, it does not give the reader a picture of the patient's performance. The objective section of the progress note is about the *patient*—it should describe the patient's response to the interventions. Examples of progress notes written by students describing what they did are found in Figure 4–3. Figure 4–4 illustrates those notes rewritten to include information about the patient's response.

Another common problem is the tendency to ramble when first learning to document. Organizing the information according to topics prevents rambling. Figure 4–5 is an example of an unorganized objective section of a progress note. Figure 4–6 is the same note, but with the information grouped by topic.

5-30-06: PT Dx: Sciatic nerve pain limiting sitting tolerance due to disc protrusion L4–5.

S: Pt. stated he has pain extending down back of Ⓡ leg, and it came on "all of a sudden" while moving his TV set. He wished he could sit long enough to watch his son's hockey games. After traction and treatment, pt. reported pain no longer in leg but located in low back.

O: Pt. demonstrated frequent wt. shifting and position changing while sitting for 15 min prior to tx. Gave mech. static lumbar traction to L4–5 area, 10 min, 90 lb, pt. prone over 1 pillow, table split, to decrease protrusion and pressure on nerve to decrease pain. Instructed pt. in ADL body mechanics, how to maintain lumbar lordosis at all times, and explained the process of a protruded disc. Instructed how to get on/off bed. Gave home instructions of McKenzie extension exercises.

A: _____

P: _____

———————————————————————————— Steven Student, SPTA/Mary Smith, PT Lic #4321

11-12-06: PT Dx: Flexed posture, shuffling gait due to Parkinson's disease.

S: Pt. states his legs feel stiff and he stumbles frequently. Feels he needs to hold on to something when he walks.

O: Pt. observed using shuffling gait with hips, knees, and trunk in slight flexion. Min. knee flexion during pre-swing and initial swing. Instructed pt. how to walk with front-wheeled rolling walker, instructed heel to toe. Did reciprocal inhibition to quads to relax quads and increase knee flexion.

A: _____

P: _____

———————————————————————————— Susan Student, SPTA/Paul Jones, PTA Lic #007

Figure 4—3 Examples of students' common mistake of writing the objective section of the progress note in terms of what they did.

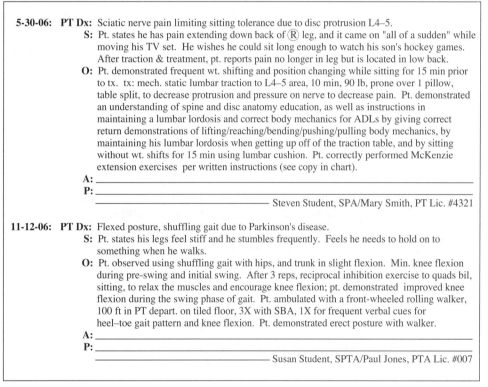

5-30-06: PT Dx: Sciatic nerve pain limiting sitting tolerance due to disc protrusion L4–5.

S: Pt. states he has pain extending down back of Ⓡ leg, and it came on "all of a sudden" while moving his TV set. He wishes he could sit long enough to watch his son's hockey games. After traction & treatment, pt. reports pain no longer in leg but is located in low back.

O: Pt. demonstrated frequent wt. shifting and position changing while sitting for 15 min prior to tx. tx: mech. static lumbar traction to L4–5 area, 10 min, 90 lb, prone over 1 pillow, table split, to decrease protrusion and pressure on nerve to decrease pain. Pt. demonstrated an understanding of spine and disc anatomy education, as well as instructions in maintaining a lumbar lordosis and correct body mechanics for ADLs by giving correct return demonstrations of lifting/reaching/bending/pushing/pulling body mechanics, by maintaining his lumbar lordosis when getting up off of the traction table, and by sitting without wt. shifts for 15 min using lumbar cushion. Pt. correctly performed McKenzie extension exercises per written instructions (see copy in chart).

A: _____

P: _____

———————————————————————————— Steven Student, SPA/Mary Smith, PT Lic. #4321

11-12-06: PT Dx: Flexed posture, shuffling gait due to Parkinson's disease.

S: Pt. states his legs feel stiff and he stumbles frequently. Feels he needs to hold on to something when he walks.

O: Pt. observed using shuffling gait with hips, and trunk in slight flexion. Min. knee flexion during pre-swing and initial swing. After 3 reps, reciprocal inhibition exercise to quads bil, sitting, to relax the muscles and encourage knee flexion; pt. demonstrated improved knee flexion during the swing phase of gait. Pt. ambulated with a front-wheeled rolling walker, 100 ft in PT depart. on tiled floor, 3X with SBA, 1X for frequent verbal cues for heel–toe gait pattern and knee flexion. Pt. demonstrated erect posture with walker.

A: _____

P: _____

———————————————————————————— Susan Student, SPTA/Paul Jones, PTA Lic. #007

Figure 4—4 The notes in Figure 4-3 written correctly in terms of what the patient did.

5-3-06:   **PT Dx:** No knee extension during gait due to biceps femoris tendon tear.
        S: Pt. states she feels more comfortable walking after US tx.
        O: Direct contact US/1 MHz/0.7 w/cm²/5 min/CW/mild heat, prone to biceps femoris insertion to increase circulation, and promote healing of tendon. Working on increasing Ⓡ knee extension for initial contact. Quadriceps, hip flexors F+ strength (F in initial eval.). Ⓡ knee AROM before tx, 20–100°, after tx 15–100°. Manual resistance strengthening exercise to quadriceps and hip flexors with isometric contractions at end of range, 10X each, 6-sec hold. Instructed in home exercises (see chart). Assessed FWB gait, no Ⓡ heel contact. Pt. correctly demonstrated home exercises.
        A: _____
        P: _____
        _____— Jim Citizen, SPTA/Tom Jones, PT Lic #1006

Figure 4—5   A disorganized objective section of the progress note in which the information rambles.

5-3-06:   **PT Dx:** No knee extension during gait due to right biceps femoris tendon tear.
        S: Pt. states she feels more comfortable walking after US tx.
        O: Pt. demonstrated FWB gait but does not fully extend right knee at initial contact. After US and exercise treatment, pt. was able consciously to improve knee extension at initial contact. Direct contact US/1MHz/0.7w/cm²/CW/mild heat, prone to right biceps femoris insertion to increase circulation, promote healing of tendon, and gain knee extension for initial contact in gait. Right quadriceps, hip flexors F+ strength (F in initial eval). Manual resistance strengthening exercise to right quads and hip flexors with isometric contractions at end of range, sitting, 10X each, 6-sec hold. Pt. correctly demonstrated home exercises to strengthen quads and hip flexors and gentle stretching exercises for hamstrings to gain knee extension during gait (see copy of written instructions in chart). Ⓡ knee AROM before tx 20–100°, after tx 15-100°.
        A: _____
        P: _____
        _____— Jim Citizen, SPTA/Tom Jones, PT Lic #1006

Figure 4—6   The note in Figure 4-5 rewritten with the information organized.

SUMMARY   The objective data content of the progress note provides proof of interventions performed, their effectiveness, and the extent of patient improvement, if any. This content must be measurable and reproducible. Objective data content includes intervention details, comparison of results of measurements and tests with previous results, visual and tactile observations made by the PTA, and descriptions of the patient's functional abilities. It should be written so the words paint a picture of the patient and the treatment session and the reader can visualize how the patient is functioning. The objective data content must be relevant to the chief complaint, the goals or functional outcomes, and the reason for the provision of skilled physical therapy services.

REFERENCES   1. Baeten, A. M., et al. (1999). *Documenting physical therapy: The reviewer perspective* (p. 41). Boston: Butterworth-Heinemann.

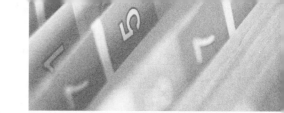

Review Exercises

1. Describe the criteria for information to be considered **objective** data.

2. List the **types** of information included in the objective data content.

3. **Describe** how results of tests and measurements are documented.

4. Explain what information should be included when describing the patient's **function.**

5. Describe what information should be included for the interventions to be **reproducible.**

6. Describe the *two* most common mistakes students make when documenting objective data.

PRACTICE EXERCISES

Practice Exercise 1 ➤ *Write "Pr" next to the problem or PT diagnosis statements, "S" next to the subjective data statements, "O" next to the objective data statements, and "N/A" if none apply.*

_____ 1. Pt. c/o pain with prolonged sitting.

_____ 2. Decubitus on sacrum measures 3 cm from Ⓛ outer edge to Ⓡ outer edge.

_____ 3. Pt. ambulates with ataxic gait, 10 ft max. assist of 2° to prevent fall.

_____ 4. Ⓡ Knee flexion PROM 30°–90°.

_____ 5. Ambulates c̄ standard walker, PWB Ⓛ bed to bathroom (20 ft), tiled surface, min. assist 1X for balance.

_____ 6. Pt. states he is fearful of crutch walking.

_____ 7. Limited ROM in Ⓛ shoulder secondary to fractured greater tubercle of humerus and unable to put on winter coat without help.

_____ 8. C/o itching in scar Ⓡ knee.

_____ 9. Transfers: supine ↔ sit c̄ min. assist of 1 for strength.

_____ 10. Unable to feed self with Ⓛ hand because of limited elbow ROM 2° Fx Ⓛ olecranon process.

_____ 11. AROM WNL bil. LEs.

_____ 12. Pt. demonstrated adequate knee flexion during initial swing c̄ verbal cueing p̄ hamstring exercises.

_____ 13. Dependent in bed mobility due to dislocated Ⓡ hip.

_____ 14. Expresses concern over lack of progress.

_____ 15. Ⓛ shoulder flexion PROM 0°–100°, lat. rot. PROM 0°–40°.

_____ 16. Kathy reports PTA courses are easy.

_____ 17. Pt. pivot transfers, NWB Ⓡ, bed ↔ w/c, max. assist 2X for strength, balance, NWB cueing.

_____ 18. Pt. rates Ⓛ knee pain 5/10 when going up stairs.

_____ 19. BP 125/80 mm Hg, pulse 78 BPM, regular, strong.

Practice Exercise 2 ➤ *Use the list of statements in Practice Exercise 1 as well as your answers to them.*

1. In the "Pr" statements, *underline* the impairment and *circle* the functional limitation.

2. In the "S" statements, *underline* the key verb that led you to write "S."

3. In the "O" statements, *underline* the key information that led you to write "O."

4. List the medical diagnoses you can find in the statements.

_____

_____

_____

_____

_____

_____

_____

_____

_____

_____

Practice Exercise 3 ➤ *Critique each of the following statements that document the results of a test or measurement. Write what is missing or incorrect, if anything, in the documentation. The first question has been answered for you to illustrate what you are to do. If the statement is fine, place an N/A in the comment section.*

The patient was able to ambulate 20 feet today.

Comment: *This statement tells the therapist how far the patient was able to ambulate but does not say anything about the patient's dependence level, equipment used, type of surface, etc. A more appropriate statement would be: The patient, with a ⓛ CVA, was able to ambulate 20 ft, 2X, with CGA and the use of a FWW on an even surface today.*

1. Mrs. Smith was able to transfer from the bed to the wheelchair, independently with SBA and verbal cueing.

   Comment: _____

   _____

   _____

   _____

2. The patient, with an L1 SCI, was able to transition from the floor to the mat.

   Comment: _____

   _____

   _____

   _____

3. Left knee flexion PROM 0°–63° in sitting position (0°–55° in initial exam).

   Comment: _____

   _____

_____

_____

4. Hip ROM 75°.

   Comment: _____

   _____

   _____

   _____

5. Hip abductor strength G- (good minus), 3/5 in initial exam.

   Comment: _____

   _____

   _____

   _____

6. Left hip hyperextension with anterior pelvic tilt, prone, 20°.

   Comment: _____

   _____

   _____

   _____

7. Circumference at right olecranon process 4 inches, upper arm 6 inches, lower arm 3 inches.

   Comment: _____

   _____

   _____

   _____

8. Blood pressure 120/70, pulse 72.

   Comment: _____

   _____

   _____

   _____

9. Circumference right wrist, supine, UE elevated 45°, 3rd metacarpal head 8 inches, 2 inches superior to 3rd metacarpal head 8 inches, superior edge of ulnar styloid process 7 cm, taken along superior border of marks.

Comment: _____

_____

_____

_____

10. Resting respiratory rate 12 breaths per minute relaxed, quiet, sitting position.

Comment: _____

_____

_____

_____

11. Left shoulder flexion 100°, abduction 100°, external rotation 60°, internal rotation 40°.

Comment: _____

_____

_____

_____

12. Left knee flexion PROM, prone with towel under thigh, 20°–110° (30°–90° initial exam).

Comment: _____

_____

_____

_____

13. Right leg 1 inch longer than left.

Comment: _____

_____

_____

_____

14. Trunk forward bend 20%.

Comment: _____

_____

_____

_____

15. Trunk side bend greater on right than left.

Comment: _____

_____

_____

_____

16. Cervical rotation to right 0°–25°, aligned with nose, sitting position, shoulders stabilized.

Comment: _____

_____

_____

_____

Practice Exercise 4 ➤ *Write each of the following objective statements in a more professional manner by using the approved abbreviations in Appendix A. The first one has been done for you.*

1. Today, the patient's blood pressure before beginning exercises was 120–70, half way through the exercise program his blood pressure was 130–80, and after cooling down from the exercise program his blood pressure was 125/75 mm Hg.

   Answer: BP ā ex 120/70 mm Hg, during ex 130/80 mm Hg, and p̄ 125/75 mm Hg.

2. Patient lacked 20 degrees of full knee extension on the right leg.

   Answer: _____

   _____

   _____

3. The patient moved from sitting in her wheelchair to standing in the parallel bars with the PTA giving the patient maximum assistance.

   Answer: _____

   _____

   _____

4. The patient was instructed in going up and down 4 steps with the axillary crutches with the handrail on the left side going up and the right side going down. The patient successfully ascended and descended the 4 steps with only verbal reminders from the PTA.

Answer: _____

_____

_____

5. The patient was placed in a side-lying position on his left side with a pillow behind his back so that ultrasound could be applied to his right shoulder.

Answer: _____

_____

_____

Practice Exercise 5 ➤ *Rewrite the following notes in the "S" and "O" sections of a SOAP note by using the abbreviations in Appendix A.*

1. Pt. is a 52-year-old female with a grade 1 MCL sprain on her right side that occurred while she was snow skiing.

S_____

O_____

2. The patient had a knee immobilizing brace on when she arrived at the clinic.

S_____

O_____

3. Patient was able to perform 3 sets of 15 ankle pumps on the right side.

S_____

O_____

4. The patient said that she cannot bend her right knee all the way yet because it is still very painful.

S_____

O_____

5. Patient was able to perform 3 sets of 10 isometric quadriceps sets on the right side.

S_____

O_____

6. Patient was able to perform 3 sets of 10 straight leg raises on the right side but complained of increased pain and needed a 3-minute rest period after completion.

S_____

O_____

7. The accident occurred 5 days ago.

S_____

O_____

8. Patient said pain was 5/10 on pain scale of 1 to 10 today when she arrived at the clinic.

S_____

O_____

9. Patient was positioned in a supine position with a pillow under her knee and given ice massage for 15 minutes to the right knee following exercises today.

S_____

O_____

10. The patient said that she and her doctor do not want to do a surgical repair unless it is absolutely necessary.

S_____

O_____

11. The patient's range of motion in the right knee is 10 to 100 degrees.

S_____

O_____

12. The patient will see the orthopedic surgeon on 9-2-06.

S_____

O_____

Practice Exercise 6 ➤   *The following goals do not follow the criteria for writing goals correctly. They do not tell the reader much about the functional outcome of the patient.*

A. *First, rewrite each goal so it contains an action (verb), can be measured, and establishes a time period for accomplishing the goal.*

B. *Second, use your imagination and rewrite each goal so it relates to a specific functional outcome or activity.*

1. Increase right knee PROM to 0°–90°.

_____

_____

_____

_____

2. Sit on edge of bed in 3 days.

_____

_____

_____

_____

3. Ambulate 30 ft using standard walker in 4 days.

_____

_____

_____

_____

4. Increase strength of hip abductors from 3/5 to 4/5.

_____

_____

_____

_____

5. Decrease pain rating on pain scale from 6/10 to 3/10.

_____

_____

_____

_____

6. Return to work.

_____

_____

_____

_____

7. Decrease pain with movement in 1 to 2 weeks.

_____

_____

_____

_____

8. Decreased edema in right thumb to allow active ROM to be WNL.

_____

_____

_____

_____

9. Able to step down a 4-inch step with no pain complaints.

_____

_____

_____

_____

10. Able to lift 10 lb from floor with 4/10 pain rating to allow occasional picking up infant son from floor in 4 weeks.

_____

_____

_____

_____

Practice Exercise 7 ➤   *The correctly written anticipated goal or expected functional outcome should have an action verb, measurable criteria for judging the quality of the performance of the action, and a time period for accomplishing the goal/outcome and should relate to a functional outcome. Critique the following goals and outcomes. Identify what is missing if a goal is not written correctly.*

1. Increase gait training to 90 ft, 4 trials, rolling walker, standby assist in 2 weeks.

   _____

   _____

   _____

2. Improve left shoulder flexion to 0°–110°.

   _____

   _____

   _____

3. Pivot transfer wheelchair to bed minimum assist.

   _____

   _____

   _____

4. Gain right ankle dorsiflexion PROM to 0°–15° in 4 weeks.

   _____

   _____

   _____

5. Ascend and descend stairs with single-end cane.

   _____

   _____

   _____

6. Strength gain in left gluteus medius in 3 weeks.

   _____

   _____

   _____

7. Transfer wheelchair to floor 3 out of 5 times in 6 weeks.

   _____

   _____

   _____

8. Ambulate independently with forearm crutches bed to dining room for all meals in 3 weeks.

_____

_____

_____

9. Lift 35-lb boxes from floor to shelf in 4 weeks.

_____

_____

_____

10. Able to perform 3 sets of 10 reps leg presses with 150 lb, consistently controlling the movement so the knees do not hyperextend and the weight plates to not clang.

_____

_____

_____

Practice Exercise 8 ▶ *Read the following progress note. Underline the subjective and objective data statements that support or provide evidence for the comments in the A section of the note.*

4-17-06 Dx: Ⓡ Colles' fracture, healed, cast removed
PT Dx: Restricted ROM in wrist with inability to open doors, limited ability to grasp and pull for dressing activities.

S: Pt. reports able to put on pantyhose today without help from husband and turned bathroom doorknob to open the door.

O: Pt. has been seen 2X. Pt. performed AROM exercises Ⓡ forearm pronation/supination while in arm whirlpool, 110°F, 20 min, to increase circulation and increase extensibility to Ⓡ wrist tissues to prepare for stretching exercises. Contract-relax stretching techniques, 5 reps each, to increase pronation, supination, and wrist extension ROM, sitting with forearm supported on table. Pt. correctly demonstrated home exercise program for strengthening finger flexion, wrist flexion and extension, and forearm pronation and supination (see copy in chart). ROM today vs. 4-10-06:

	4-17-06	4-10-06
Ⓡ pronation	0°–50°	0°–40°
Ⓡ supination	0°–70°	0°–60°
Wrist extension	0°–30°	0°–20°

Grip strength 20 lb today, 10 lb 4-10-06. Pt. turned door handles and opened all inside doors in the clinic using Ⓡ hand but unable to turn handle and open door to outside. Able to grasp rope on scale and pull, exerting 3-lb force (2-lb 4-10-06).

A: Strengthening and stretching treatment procedures effective in increasing strength and ROM, improving progress toward goals of independent dressing activities and ability to open all types of doors.

P: To see pt. on 4-24-06 and notify PT discharge eval to be 4-31-06. Will work on opening outside doors next visit.

—Sally Citizen, PTA, Lic. 5631

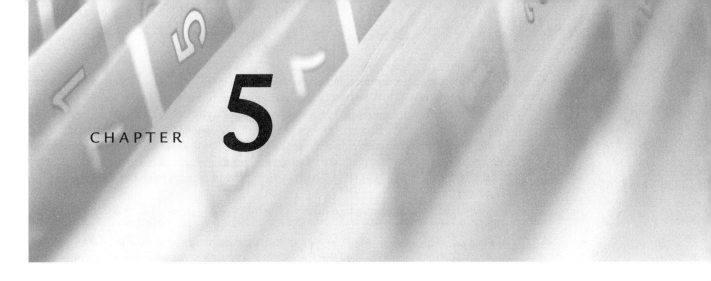

CHAPTER **5**

What Is Assessment Data and Why It Is Important

LEARNING OBJECTIVES

After studying this chapter, the student will be able to:

☐ Identify assessment data.

☐ Organize assessment data for easy reading and understanding.

☐ Demonstrate adherence to recommended guidelines for documenting assessment data.

☐ Document the patient's functional abilities to provide the reader with a picture of patient's functional level and rate of progression.

☐ Document interventions so they are reproducible by another PTA or a PT.

☐ Document assessment data consistent with the data in the PT's initial examination.

☐ Identify common mistakes students typically make when documenting assessment data.

☐ Explain the difference between subjective, objective, and assessment information.

INTRODUCTION

The "*A*" stands for *assessment*. In this section of the evaluation report, the PT summarizes the subjective and objective information and answers the question, "What does it mean?" In the assessment section, the PT also interprets, makes a clinical judgment, and sets functional outcomes and goals on the basis of the information in the subjective and objective sections. In the progress note, the PTA summarizes the information in the subjective and objective sections and reports the progress being made toward accomplishing the goals in the assessment sections. The PTA's summary also answers the "what does it mean?" question.

After reviewing subjective and objective data, the informative facts, a person reading the medical record may ask, "What does it mean?" Readers of the record who are not trained in physical therapy (e.g., insurance representatives, lawyers, physicians) may not understand the subjective and objective data unless they are interpreted. The interpretation and significance of the subjective and objective data are reflected in the initial evaluation report, the physical therapy diagnosis, the treatment plan and goals, and the treatment outcomes and effectiveness. These elements of the record support the necessity for the physical therapy medical treatment.

The PTA documents the significance of the data in the progress note by describing the patient's response to the treatment plan and the patient's progress toward the accomplishment of the goals. This information is located in the A (assessment) section of the SOAP outline, the E (evaluation) section of the DEP format, and the problems and functional outcome goals portions of the FOR. This information is addressed throughout the PSPG-organized progress note: the physical therapy diagnosis or problem constitutes the first P (problem) section, the rationale for modified treatment plans contained in the second P (plan) section is based on the significance of the data presented in the assessment section, and the discussion about progress toward goals is provided in the G section. For ease of discussion in this chapter, this information will be referred to as interpretation of the data content. Interpretation of the data content is more complex in the PT's evaluation reports than in the PTA's progress notes.

ASSESSMENT DATA

Assessment data consists of information about the patient's progress, treatment effectiveness, completion of goals set by the PT in the initial evaluation, changes recommended in the plan of care, and goals completed for the individual treatment sessions. The PTA is responsible for communicating any recommended changes in the plan of care, completion of skills within the goals set by the PT, recommendations for changes within the plan of care, and recommendations for discharge.

Goals or Functional Outcomes

INITIAL EXAMINATION: Goals or functional outcomes are set by the patient and PT during the initial evaluation.

PROGRESS NOTE: Goals may need to be modified as the patient and the PTA become better acquainted and the PTA learns more about the patient's needs and desires. See the following example.

> Sam told the PT that he needs to be able to climb only two steps to get into his house; the rest of his house is on one floor. They set a stair-climbing goal: "To be able to climb two steps independently using the railing on the left and be able to ascend and descend a curb independently with no ambulation device." One week later, during a treatment session, Sam is telling Jim about his cabin on a nearby lake and how anxious he is to go to the cabin and go fishing. Sam casually mentions that there are six wooden steps down to the dock. Jim makes a mental note and also documents in the patient's medical record to share this information with the PT and to suggest that the goal be modified.

Response to Treatment

PROGRESS NOTE: Reporting the patient's ability to perform the prescribed treatment documents the effectiveness of the treatment program and influences future treatment plans. See the following example:

> PTA Brenda treats Robert, who has a mild lumbar disc protrusion and complains of waking up often in the night with tingling in his left leg. During yesterday's treatment session, Brenda showed Robert how to use pillows and a rolled towel to support his spine and maintain proper positioning while sleeping. Today, Robert reports that he awoke only three times last night because of back soreness and didn't have any tingling in his leg. Brenda makes a mental note to quote Robert in the subjective section of the progress note to provide evidence that her instructions in sleeping positions were effective and to adapt the treatment plan (following communication with the PT) to reflect goals towards strengthening and increased range of motion.

Level of Function in the Initial Examination

INITIAL EXAMINATION: The initial examination describes the patient's functional level at the time of the examination.

PROGRESS NOTE: The patient's description of his or her functional level may help the PTA assess the patient's progress or response to treatment. See the following example:

> PTA Mary is treating Mr. Jones, who had an acute flare-up of osteoarthritis in his hands. His chief complaint during the initial evaluation was an inability to dress himself, especially handling buttons and snaps, because of the pain. Today he arrives wearing a sweater, which he said he buttoned without needing to ask for help. This comment may be evidence in the progress note that Mr. Jones has met a goal or outcome and should be documented accordingly.

ORGANIZING ASSESSMENT DATA

The assessment information, in the initial examination report, may be more complex and detailed than the assessment information in the progress notes. The PT may organize this information into subcategories, such as active and passive range of motion, strength, alignment, presence of any abnormal reflexes or responses, muscle tone, quality of movement, automatic reactions and balance responses, functional capabilities such as transition in and out of different positions and ability to walk on even and uneven surfaces, ability to ascend and descend steps, the patient's functional outcomes for improvement in activity, and the function and reduction of any perceived pain. It is also important to address any need for adaptive equipment at this time. This helps the PT confine the data to only the categories that are relevant. Organizing the content makes it easy to read and to locate information. The example in Figure 5–1 presents assessment data that is not necessarily supported by the subjective and objective portions of the note. In Figure 5–2, the note presents assessment information that does not include the goals.

A. Situation: Patient had stroke (CVA) 2 weeks ago and is now home, receiving physical therapy 3 times a week through a home health agency. His wife is the caregiver.

Dx: Ⓡ CVA.

PT Dx: Ⓛ hemiparesis with dependent mobility in all aspects.

Expected functional outcomes: At anticipated discharge date in 1 month.
1. Patient will ambulate with an assistive device and minimal assist for balance to the bathroom and to meals in 3 weeks.
2. Patient will be able to manage two steps with an assistive device and a railing as well as car transfers for next visit to the doctor in 4 weeks.

Anticipated goals:
1. Pt. will consistently move up and down in bed and roll from side to side with SBA in 2 weeks.
2. Pt. will consistently roll to Ⓛ side and reach for telephone and call bell with SBA in 3 weeks.
3. Pt. will consistently move from supine to sitting on edge of bed and return to supine position with minimal assist to help swing Ⓛ leg into bed in 1 week.
4. Pt. will consistently move from sitting to standing and back to sitting from bed, toilet, wheelchair, and standard chair with minimum assist for balance, control, and even weight-bearing cueing in 2 weeks.
5. Using a quad cane, pt. will consistently ambulate bed to bathroom, and to meals with moderate assist for balance control and gait posture cueing in 1 week.

B. Situation: Patient is 1 week postoperation for total hip replacement and is in a subacute rehabilitation unit. Patient is receiving physical therapy 2X/day with plans to be discharged to home.

Dx: Ⓛ total hip replacement

PT Dx: Weakened hip musculature and dependent in rising from sit to stand and ambulation.

Expected functional outcomes: At anticipated discharge in 20 days, patient will transfer and ambulate independently for return to home.
1. Patient will independently and consistently move from sit to stand and stand to sit using elevated toilet seat, and all other surfaces no lower than 18 inches.
2. Patient will independently and consistently walk with a straight cane on all surfaces and in the community.

Anticipated goals:
1. Pt. will consistently be able to sit to stand and return with SBA if boost is needed from edge of bed, elevated toilet seat, wheelchair, and standard dining room chair in 10 days.
2. Pt. will consistently be able to ambulate using a straight cane for balance on tiled and carpeted level surfaces, to bathroom and dining room for meals with SBA for balance control in 10 days.

Figure 5—1 Progress note with assessment statements that are not supported by information in subjective or objective data, or both.

3-6-06   **Dx:** (R) UE lymphedema 2° mastectomy.
   PT Dx: Edema (R) UE limiting elbow ROM with inability to feed self and groom hair using (R) UE.
Pt. states she is able to move her arm and use it more to help dress herself and to adjust her bed covers.
Measurements taken before and after ICP/1 hr/50 lb/30 sec on 10 sec off/supine/(R) UE elevated 45° to
reduce edema. ⎯⎯⎯⎯⎯⎯⎯⎯⎯⎯⎯⎯⎯⎯⎯⎯⎯⎯⎯⎯⎯⎯⎯

	Before	After	3-4-06
Superior edge olecranon process	13"	12"	14"
3" above edge olecranon process	13.5"	12.5"	14.5"
3" below edge olecranon process	12.5"	11.5"	13.5"

All measurements read at superior edge of mark. Elbow flexion 0–95° today compared with 0–85° on
3-4-06. Observed pt. feeding self today using long-handled spoon in (R) hand. ICP effective in reducing
edema and allowing increased ROM in elbow flexion. Pt. making progress toward goal of decreased edema
and increased elbow room so pt. wil be independent in feeding and grooming hair without needing assistive
devices. Will continue ICP treatment per PT initial plan.

Richard Student, SPTA/JimTherapist, PT Lic #1063

Figure 5–2   A progress note that does not mention the goals but confines comments only to the data that
measure the impairment severity level and the treatment procedures.

WRITING ASSESSMENT DATA

The APTA's *Guidelines for Physical Therapy Documentation* state that the evaluation report
should include the physical therapy diagnosis or problem and the goals to be accomplished.[1]
When organizing the evaluation information in SOAP format, the PT places this information
in the A section. This section contains the PT's interpretation of the signs and symptoms, test
results, and observations made during the examination, as well as a conclusion or judgment
about the meaning or relevance of the information. The physical therapy diagnoses are based
on this interpretation. Desired functional outcomes and anticipated goals are based on the
problems. Thus, the subjective and objective information is summarized, and the "what does
it mean?" question is answered in the assessment section of the SOAP note.

The Physical Therapy Diagnosis/Problem

The first conclusion the PT reaches after evaluating the data is the identification of the physical therapy diagnosis or problem (see Chapter 2). It is necessary to determine this information to develop an appropriate plan of care that addresses the patient's decreased level of
function and that restores the patient to the highest level of function following skilled therapeutic intervention.

Outcomes and Goals

The PT and the patient (or a representative of the patient) collaborate to establish the expected
functional outcomes and anticipated goals for the duration of the physical therapy treatment.
The *Guide to Physical Therapist Practice* indicates that **goals** generally address impairments
and **outcomes** relate to the patient's functional limitations or reason he or she is receiving
therapy.[2]

Expected Functional Outcomes

The expected functional outcome is a broad statement describing the functional abilities necessary for the patient to no longer require physical therapy. **Functional abilities** are the abilities to perform activities or tasks that support the individual's physical, social, and
psychological well-being, creating a personal sense of meaningful living.[2] When these abilities are regained, the patient's functional limitations and the disability identified in the physical therapy diagnosis or problem will be eliminated or decreased in severity. This is the
criterion for the conclusion of the episode of physical therapy care. The *Guide to Physical
Therapist Practice* defines **episode of physical therapy care** as: "All physical therapy services that are (1) provided by a physical therapist or under the direction and supervision of a
physical therapist, (2) provided in an unbroken sequence, and (3) related to the physical therapy interventions for a given condition or problem . . ."[2]

During a patient's episode of care, he or she may transfer to another facility (perhaps
more than once) to receive a continuum of physical therapy services. Outcomes may be developed that describe the functional abilities the patient will need to accomplish to be discharged
from one facility and be transferred to the next. These short-term outcomes are the steps that
must be complete to accomplish the expected functional outcome.

For example, the patient who has undergone total knee-replacement surgery desires to return to independence in walking throughout her home and in the community. This becomes the expected functional outcome for this patient's episode of physical therapy care. The hospital physical therapist works toward the short-term outcome of independent ambulation with a walker in bedroom, bathroom, and short distances in the hall. When the patient is transferred to a rehabilitation facility, therapy is directed toward the short-term outcome of independent ambulation with an appropriate ambulation aid for longer distances and on carpeting, grass, gravel, stairs, and ramps.

When this is accomplished, the patient is discharged and transferred to home where the home health-care therapist works toward the expected functional outcome for this episode of care, independent ambulation without an ambulation aid in the home and community.

Anticipated Goals

Anticipated goals describe the changes in the impairments necessary for the patient's function to improve. They are the steps for accomplishing the outcomes and thus should relate to the outcomes. For example, goals may describe the desired strength gain, range of motion improvement, and balance improvement needed for the outcome to be accomplished. They may describe the progression of the quality of the movement, the efficiency of the task, and the assist needed to eventually accomplish the functional outcome.

Writing the Functional Outcomes and Goals

Outcomes and goals must be written to include the **action or performance** (e.g., will ambulate), the **measurable criteria** that determine whether a task has been accomplished (e.g., walked from bedroom to kitchen), and a **time period** within which it is expected the outcome or goal will be met (e.g., in 1 week). Measurable criteria are the most important part of the outcome and goal. An action or performance can be measured in a variety of ways. A few examples of measurable criteria are strength grade, degrees of joint motion, scores on standardized test, seconds/minutes, description of the quality of the movement, proper posture/body mechanics, correct techniques, amount of assist needed, assistive equipment needed, and pain rating. When goals address specific impairments, they should also describe how the desired change in the impairment relates to the desired change in the functional limitation. A description of the change in function becomes another method of measuring the accomplishment of the goal. *A description of the change in function becomes the best measurement to ensure third-party reimbursement.* Examples of expected functional outcomes and anticipated goals are given in Figure 5–3. Writing the outcomes and goals in this manner gives the PTA direction for planning treatment sessions that include activities enabling the patient's progression toward the goal, methods for measuring the patient's progress, and standards for determining when to recommend termination of treatment.

Examples of goals relating to the desired change in the impairments and functional limitations include the following:

- ROM for left shoulder flexion will improve 0°–110° so patient can reach top of head for grooming in 2 weeks.

10-25-06   Dx: Ⓡ CVA.
    PT Dx: Ⓛ hemiparesis with dependent mobility in all aspects.
Pt. has been receiving PT twice a day for 3 days. Pt. able to lift buttocks with smooth motion 5X & scoot up and down in bed, roll 5X independently to Ⓛ side, roll to Ⓡ side with minimum assist to bring Ⓛ shoulder over 5X. Pt. practiced 3X moving from sitting on edge of bed to sidelying on three pillows and returned to sitting with minimum assist to initiate sidelying to sit 1X. Able to move from sit to stand and to return to sit from edge of bed with bed raised to highest level, SBA for cueing for even wt. bearing, 3X. Pt. ambulated from bed to bathroom to bed 3X using quad cane and moderate assist for balance and assist in advancing Ⓛ leg 2X. Pt. circumducts Ⓛ leg due to inability to flex knee during pre-swing. Pt. making progress toward goals of independent bed mobility, sit to stand with SBA and ambulation with quad cane and minimum assist. Will consult with PT about adding exercises for knee flexion with hip extended to improve gait next session. Jane Doe, PTA Lic. #2961

Figure 5—3   Examples of expected functional outcomes and anticipated goals.

- Strength of right gluteus medius will increase to 4/5 so patient will no longer demonstrate a significant trunk shift to the right during stance phase of ambulation in 4 weeks.
- Amount of edema will decrease so girth measurements of right upper arm will be within 1 inch of left upper arm and patient's right arm will fit into the sleeves of her clothing in 1 week.

In the first goal, the action or performance is improvement in shoulder flexion, the measurable criteria are ROM 0°–110° and the patient's ability to reach the top of his head, and the time period is 2 weeks.

In the second goal, the action or performance is increased strength, the measurable criteria are 4/5-strength grade and no demonstration of a significant trunk shift to the right, and the time period is 4 weeks. The reader should determine whether the third goal is properly written.

The PTA helping the patient to accomplish the first goal sees that the desired improvement in flexion needs to be met in 2 weeks. The PTA can plan each treatment session to include appropriate exercises and activities that will increase the flexion range of motion. The PTA will guide the exercises accordingly, monitoring progress by measuring the range of motion, and observing the patient's attempts to touch the top of his head. At 2 weeks, the goal is that the patient is able to perform left shoulder flexion through the range of motion from 0°–110° and reach the top of his head. The PTA can report to the PT and record achievement of the goal in the progress note.

The anticipated goals shown in Figure 5–3 also contain the qualities that demonstrate proper formulation and writing. In **Situation A**, the performance goals are moving up and down in bed, rolling from side to side, and reaching for the telephone and call bell. The measurable criterion is standby assist, and the time period is 2 weeks. In this case, the PTA can structure the treatment sessions to include instructions and practice in bed mobility, rolling, and reaching for the telephone and call bell. The PTA will help the patient progress by decreasing the amount of assistance provided until the patient can perform these movements with standby assist. In **Situation B**, the PTA will work with the patient to improve the patient's ability to move from supine to a sitting position on the edge of the bed (action). The PTA will help the patient progress by decreasing the level of assistance provided until only minimal assist is needed (measurable criterion). The PTA may choose to spend most of the treatment session time on this activity during the first week, because the time period for meeting this goal is just 1 week. These goals describe functional tasks and do not include other impairments, so a description of the patient performing the tasks with standby assist is the only measurable criterion needed. Goals could be written to include the quality of the movements or speed of the movement as other measurable criteria for these functional tasks.

Although the PTA does not design the functional outcomes or the anticipated goals, he or she can work with the PT by offering suggestions, notifying the PT when goals are met, and recognizing when the PT needs to modify or change goals. A PTA may write goals for each treatment *session* to help the PTA stay focused on the progression of the patient toward accomplishing the anticipated goals and the functional outcomes. **The treatment *session* goals are the steps to accomplish the anticipated goals set by the physical therapist.**

The PTA knows the patient's evaluation results and refers to the goals listed in the evaluation when writing the interpretation of the progress note data. This coordination of the evaluation and the progress note provides written proof of the PT–PTA team approach to the patient's care, thus enabling the reader to determine the quality of care being provided.

INTERPRETATION OF THE DATA CONTENT IN THE PROGRESS NOTE

Interpretation of the data is the most important section of the progress note. Most readers of the medical record look for this information first *because it tells the reader whether the physical therapy care is helping the patient*. It is the PTA's summary of the progress note data with comments about the relevance and meaning of the information. These comments inform the reader of the patient's response to the treatment plan. This is in contrast to the objective section, which records the patient's response to each intervention. The reader of the progress note is told whether the patient is making progress toward accomplishing the outcomes and goals. Any comment made by the PTA must be supported by the subjective and/or objective information. The comments should be grouped or organized so the information is easy to follow and understand.

Change in the Impairment

A summary of the meaning of measurements and test results or observations recorded in the objective data can describe a change in the impairment severity when this information is compared with the status of the patient at the initial evaluation. For example, if the objective data include girth measurements of the patient's arm that are less than previous measurements and the patient's elbow flexion measurements show greater range of motion, the PTA can comment that the intervention has been effective in decreasing the swelling and thus improving the ability of the elbow to move (decreasing the severity of the impairment). See the example progress note in Figure 5–4.

Progress Towards Functional Outcomes and Goals

The PTA informs the reader about the patient's progress through comments about improvement in functional abilities and progress toward or accomplishment of the expected functional outcomes and anticipated goals. A statement about whether an outcome or goal has been met is documented in this section. The reader also can find a description of the patient's functioning in the objective data, which will provide evidence to support the PTA's conclusion about progress toward the outcome or goal (Fig. 5–5).

Lack of Progress Towards Goals

Lack of progress or ineffectiveness of an intervention or the treatment plan is acknowledged, and comments are made about the complicating factors. The PTA may offer suggestions and indicate the need to consult the PT. Again, there should be subjective or objective information to substantiate the PTA's conclusion or opinion. Figure 5–6 is an example of a progress note reporting lack of progress and offering recommendations.

Inconsistency in the Data

Sometimes there is an inconsistency between the subjective information and the objective information. The PTA calls the reader's attention to this in the interpretation of the data content. For example, a patient may report a pain rating of 9 on a scale of 1 to 10, 10 meaning excruciating pain. The PTA may observe the patient moving about in a relaxed manner, using smooth movements with no demonstration of pain behaviors or mannerisms. This inconsistency is noted, and the PTA may want to include possible suggestions as to what to do. Again, this is a good place for consultation with the PT (Fig. 5–7). The PTA should be cautious when documenting inconsistencies, because this information may be interpreted as accusing the patient of lying or faking the injury or illness. The subjective and objective data should indicate clearly that something "isn't right." The PTA should also confirm the inconsistency when interpreting the data. The inconsistency may indicate that the patient should be referred to another health-care provider or have the treatment plan revised.

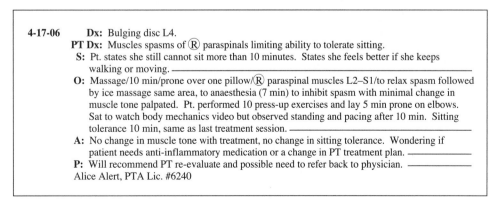

Figure 5–4 Example of progress note describing a change in the impairment severity.

3-19-06 PT Dx: Anterior rotation of right ilium limiting sitting and stair climbing tolerance. Patient states she has been doing her home exercises regularly, can sit 45 minutes now, but still has pain when attempting to step up with her right leg. Reports feeling unsafe when carrying her 18-month-old daughter up the stairs. Rates her pain 7/10 before and after treatment. Pt. has been seen for three sessions. Direct contact US/1 MHz/vigorous heat/10 min/prone/right PSIS/to relax muscle spasms and prepare ligaments for mobilization. Pt. correctly performed muscle energy self-mobilization techniques to move ilium posteriorly. (See copy of instructions in chart.) Equal leg length observed supine and long sitting after US & mobilization, uneven leg length during same test before tx. Unable to palpate muscle spasms or level of PSIS due to patient's obesity. Patient correctly demonstrated her home exercises (see copy in chart), and used correct body mechanics to minimize right hip flexion when reviewing safe technique for picking up her baby. Ambulates with an antalgic limp, shorter step length and stance time on the right. Unable to step up on 7-inch stair with right leg, due to reporting too much pain. Sat with good posture, relaxed, minimal weight shifting 45 minutes watching nutrition video and waiting for her "ride." As patient was leaving the clinic, observed her climbing into her pick-up truck by stepping up with her right leg and using smooth, quick movements. This looked like it required approximately 80–90° hip flexion. Goal of 45-minute sitting tolerance met. Progress toward outcome of safe stair climbing without railing and using step-over-step pattern appears 0% in the clinic. Performance in the clinic of good sitting tolerance but poor stair climbing tolerance is inconsistent with patient's pain rating, equal leg length test, and observed performance outside the clinic. Will consult PT as to what should be done next treatment session. Pt. has two more treatment sessions scheduled. Puzzled Assistant, PTA Lic. #439

Figure 5—5   Evidence in the data that supports the PTA's conclusion about progress toward the goal.

1-17-06 PT Dx: Decreased walking tolerance due to Ⓡ quad tendon repair.
   S: Pt. states eager to walk with cane, no c/o. _____
   O: tx: Respond E-stim./distal end Ⓡ quad/supine/15 min/motor response/for muscle re-education. Pt. performed three sets of 15 reps of each of following strengthening exercises in supine: quad sets, terminal knee extensions, AROM hip abd./add., SLR. Pt. ambulated 150 ft from bed down hall, tiled level surface, with single end cane in Ⓛ UE, contact guard assist for sense of balance and security. _____
   A: Decreased quad strength, decreased control with knee extension ex. Concern with problem of no superior excursion with max. attempt of quad set. At max. attempt, patella is able to be shifted med. & lat. Suspicion of scarring & adhesion on Ⓡ quad tendon. _____
   P: More balance work with SEC. Cont. tx 3X/week. Will consult PT about patella concerns. Pt. will see physician at 1st of next week. Mary Smith, PTA Lic. #346

Figure 5—6   An example of a progress note in which lack of progress is reported and recommendations are made.

3-5-06   Dx: Fx Ⓡ humerus, cast removed 3-3-06.
   PT Dx: Limited elbow ROM with inability to reach above second button from top, face, or hair.
      S: Pt. states his arm seems to be getting stronger, as he can lift a 5-lb bucket of water. _____

O: Elbow ROM:	**before tx**	**after tx**
flexion	40–115°	37–119°
pronation/supination	0–10° both	0–14°

All other UE ROMs WNL. _____

Skin that was under cast still dry and flaking, color WNL, no pressure areas evident. Wlp/102°F/20 min/Ⓡ UE/to relax arm muscles, débride dry skin, and prepare for exercise. Pt. performed AROM exercises per instructions,10 reps each elbow flex/ext, forearm pronation/supination in water during last 10 min of treatment. Following wlp, pt. correctly demonstrated home exercise program to increase elbow ROM and strength (see copy in chart). _____
      A: Moist heat and exercise effective in increasing elbow ROM.
      P: Will consult PT about discontinuing whirlpool after tomorrow's session and will progress difficulty of exercises. Four more tx sessions scheduled.
                              Jim Jones, SPTA/Mary Therapist, PT (Lic. #007)

Figure 5—7   Documentation of inconsistent information in the data with reference to PT consultation.

Common Student Mistakes When Documenting the Interpretation of the Data Content

Comments such as "pt. tolerated treatment well" and "pt. was cooperative and motivated" are commonly found in documentation. These types of comments are to be avoided unless they are relevant to the content of the entire progress note and are supported by the subjective and objective data. This information is better presented through descriptions and measurements of the patient's response and functional abilities.

Students commonly comment about something that is not mentioned previously in the note. Sometimes a topic is documented that appears to "come out of nowhere." Again, evidence in the subjective or objective data must be present to support the interpretation of the data. Figure 5–1 is an example of a note with information that is not supported by data in the note.

It is not unusual to see students' notes that do not mention the goals or provide any comments about whether the patient is accomplishing the outcomes or goals. Comments tend to be only about the data that measure the impairment severity level and about the treatment procedures. Figure 5–2 illustrates this type of mistake.

SUMMARY

The interpretation of the data portion of the PTA progress note provides a summary of the subjective and objective information, thereby making the data meaningful. Comments are made about the patient's progress and the effectiveness of the treatment plan. This section must always contain statements describing the patient's progress toward accomplishing the outcomes and goals listed in the initial evaluation. It coordinates the initial evaluation with the progress notes to demonstrate PT–PTA communication, teamwork, and continuum of care. The PTA may make suggestions and report information that should be brought to the PT's attention.

All statements in this section must be supported by the subjective or objective information. The same rules previously discussed about subjective and objective content also apply. Topics in this section should be organized and easy to read. All information must be relevant to the treatment plan and the patient's problem.

REFERENCES

1. American Physical Therapy Association. (June 2003). Guidelines for physical therapy documentation. In *Guide to physical therapist practice* (2nd ed.). Alexandria, VA: APTA.
2. American Physical Therapy Association. (June 2003). Documentation for physical therapist patient/client management. In *Guide to physical therapist practice* (2nd ed.). Alexandria, VA: APTA.

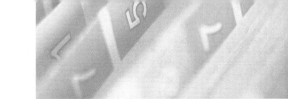

Review Exercises

1. **Define** assessment data.

2. Discuss the **type** of assessment data relevant to the patient that should be included in the progress note by the PTA.

3. Describe the **organization** of assessment data.

4. Who is involved in the establishment of the expected functional outcomes and anticipated goals for the PT treatment?

5. Explain **why** information about range of motion is assessment data.

6. Discuss **two** mistakes students often make when writing assessment data.

PRACTICE EXERCISES

Practice Exercise 1 ➤ *Write "Pr" next to statements that describe the physical therapy problem or diagnosis, "S" next to statements that fit the subjective data category, "O" next to the statements that fit the objective data category, and "A" next to the statements that fit the assessment data category.*

1. _____ Pt. states she has a clear understanding of her disease and her prognosis.

2. _____ Pt. expresses surprise that the ice massage relaxed her muscle spasm.

3. _____ Muscle spasms Ⓛ lumbar paraspinals with sitting tolerance limited to 10 min.

4. _____ Pt. describes tingling pain down back of Ⓡ leg to heel.

5. _____ Dependent in ADLs because of flaccid paralysis in Ⓡ upper and lower extremities.

6. _____ Sue states her Ⓛ ear hurts.

7. _____ Pt. able to reach above head to comb hair independently with return of full AROM in shoulder.

8. _____ Reports he must be able to return to work as a welder.

9. _____ Patient states the doctor told her she had a laceration in her Ⓡ vastus medialis.

10. _____ Paraplegic 2° SCI T12 and dependent in wheelchair transfers.

11. _____ States Hx of RA since 1980.

12. _____ Pt. denies pain c̄ cough.

13. _____ States injury occurred December 31, 1999.

14. _____ SPTA c/o he has to sit for 2 hours in the PTA lectures.

15. _____ Pt. grip strength has increased and she is now able to turn all doorknobs independently.

16. _____ Describes his pain as "burning."

17. _____ Unable to sit because of decubitus over sacrum.

18. _____ Unable to feed self because of limited elbow flexion.

19. _____ Pt. rates her pain a 4 on an ascending scale of 1–10.

20. _____ States able to sit through a 2-hour movie last night.

Practice Exercise 2 ➤ *Follow the directions in each question.*

1. For the statements in Practice Exercise 1 to which you answered "Pr," <u>underline</u> the impairment and <u>circle</u> the functional limitation.

2. For the statements in Practice Exercise 1 to which you answered "S," <u>underline</u> the verb in the statement that clued you in to this being a subjective statement.

3. List the medical diagnoses you can find in the statements.

4. Identify any statements that denote an "assessment" of the patient.

_____

_____

_____

_____

_____

Practice Exercise 3 ➤ *You are treating Nancy, who has been diagnosed as having a mild disc protrusion at L4,5 with spasms in the right lumbar paraspinal muscles. You read in the PT initial examination/evaluation that she reported pain in the right lower back and buttock areas, and you see the areas marked on a body drawing. The spasms and pain have interfered with Nancy's ability to sit; she is unable to tolerate sitting longer than 15 minutes and unable to sleep more than 2 hours at a time. She also reports having difficulty with bathing and dressing activities. Nancy works as a nursing assistant at the local hospital and has been unable to perform her job tasks. The desired functional outcomes for Nancy are to be able to sit 30 minutes, sleep 5 hours, achieve independence in bathing and dressing, and return to her work as a nursing assistant. The treatment plan and objectives are to include massage to the lumbar paraspinal muscles to relax the spasms, static pelvic traction for 10 minutes to encourage receding of the disc protrusion and stretching and relaxing the lumbar paraspinal muscles, patient education in a home exercise program for lumbar extension and control of the disc protrusion, and instructions on posture and body mechanics for correct and safe sitting, sleeping, bathing, dressing, and performance of work tasks. You have written this progress note:*

6-3-00: Dx: Disc protrusion L4,5.
  PT Dx: Muscle spasms lumbar paraspinals with limited sitting, sleeping tolerance, difficulty with ADLs, and unable to perform work tasks.

Patient states she was able to sit through 30 minutes of *The Young and The Restless* soap opera yesterday. Rates her pain a 5 on an ascending scale of 1–10. Patient has received 4 treatment sessions. Decrease in muscle tone palpable after 10-minute massage to right lumbar paraspinal muscles, prone position over one thin pillow. Unable to tolerate lying propped on elbows because of pain before traction, able to lie propped on elbows 5 minutes following 10 minutes, prone, static pelvic traction, 70 pounds. No pain in buttock area. Correctly performed lumbar extension exercises 1, 2, and 3 of home exercise program (see copy in chart) and observed consistently using correct sitting posture with lumbar roll. Patient required frequent verbal cueing for correct body mechanics while performing 10 repetitions (3 reps in initial eval.) of circuit of job simulation activities consisting of bed making, rolling, and moving 30 pounds (10 pounds in initial eval.) dummy "patient" in bed, pivot transferring the dummy, and wheelchair handling. She did 10 back arches between each task without reminders. Patient has reached 30-minute sitting tolerance outcome, is independent with home exercise program, and compliant with techniques for controlling the protrusion. Progress toward outcome of return to work is 60% with more consistent use of correct body mechanics and ability to lift 50-pound dummy required. Patient to continue treatment sessions 3X/week for 2 more weeks per PT's initial plan. Will notify PT that interim evaluation is scheduled for 6-7-00.

—Sue Smith, PTA, Lic. 0003

Describe what the PTA has done incorrectly in writing this note and rewrite it correctly.

_____

_____

_____

_____

_____

_____

_____

_____

_____

_____

_____

Practice Exercise 4 ➤   *Place "Yes" next to relevant assessment data statements and "No" next to those that do not seem relevant.*

_____ 1. Client stated her dog was hit by a car last night and she felt too depressed today to do her exercises.

_____ 2. Client reported he progressed his exercises to 50 push-ups yesterday.

_____ 3. Patient was able to ambulate independently, 50 ft with FFW walker.

_____ 4. Patient states he does not like the hospital food and is hungry for some Dairy Queen.

_____ 5. Patient was able to lift 5 lb in shoulder flexion 10X, 3 sets, today.

_____ 6. Patient states she is now able to reach the second shelf of her kitchen cupboard to reach for a glass.

_____ 7. Patient is able to walk 100 ft, independently, 2X.

_____ 8. Client reports experiencing an aching in his "elbow bone" after the ultrasound treatment yesterday.

_____ 9. Patient says she has 10 grandchildren and 4 great grandchildren.

_____ 10. Client states she forgot to tell the PT that she loves to bowl.

_____ 11. Patient is able to move from sit to stand, independently, with fair balance, 4X.

_____ 12. Client reports he sat in his fishing boat 3 hours and caught a 7-pound Northern Pike this weekend.

_____ 13. Client states he played golf yesterday for the first time since his back injury.

_____ 14. Patient can ambulate 25 ft with wheeled walker and standby assist.

_____ 15. Client states she cannot turn her head to look over her shoulder to back the car out of the garage.

_____ 16. Patient's mother wants to know when her son will come out of the coma.

_____ 17. Patient can lift 20 lb in hip flexion, 10X, 2 sets.

_____ 18. Patient describes his flight of stairs with 10 steps, a landing, then 5 more steps and the railing on the right when going up.

_____ 19. Patient is able to ascend and descend 4 steps with the use of her cane and one rail to get in and out of her apartment with CGA.

_____ 20. Patient states, "I'm going to Macy's to shop and have lunch today." (Patient is 89 years old and is a resident in a long-term-care facility in a small town in Ohio. She has been placed on some new medication.)

Practice Exercise 5 ➤ *The progress notes in Figure 4–4 in Chapter 4 are incomplete. Finish the notes by writing the assessment sections, stating what you will do next.*

_____

_____

_____

_____

_____

_____

_____

_____

_____

Practice Exercise 6 ➤ *The progress note in Figure 4–6 in Chapter 4 is incomplete. Finish the note by writing the assessment section, stating what you will do next.*

_____

_____

_____

_____

_____

_____

_____

Practice Exercise 7 ➤   *Read the objectives in the Practice Exercise 7 in Chapter 4 listed below. Circle the activity or intervention and underline the measurable information. An example is given. Then provide the frequencies and durations (time periods) for each objective on the blank lines.*

⌐Ultra Sound⌐ to Ⓡ trochanteric bursa, moderate heating effect, to increase circulation to <u>decrease inflammation and discomfort</u>.

1. Increase gait training to 90 feet, 4 trials, rolling walker, standby assist in 2 weeks.

    _____

    _____

2. Improve left shoulder flexion to 0°–110°.

    _____

    _____

3. Pivot transfer wheelchair to bed, minimum assist.

    _____

    _____

4. Gain right ankle dorsiflexion PROM to 0°–15°.

    _____

    _____

5. Ascend and descend stairs with single-end cane.

    _____

    _____

6. Strength gain in left gluteus medius in 3 weeks.

    _____

    _____

7. Transfer wheelchair to floor 3 out of 5 times in 6 weeks.

    _____

    _____

8. Ambulate independently with forearm crutches from bed to dining room for all meals in 3 weeks.

    _____

    _____

9. Lift 35-lb boxes from floor to shelf in 4 weeks.

_____

_____

10. Able to perform 3 sets of 10 reps leg presses with 150 lb, consistently controlling the movement so the knees do not hyperextend and the weight plates do not clang.

_____

_____

Practice Exercise 8 ➤ *Look at Figure 5–1. It illustrates documentation of information in the A section of this SOAP-organized note that is not mentioned in the subjective or objective sections. There is more in this note that does not constitute quality documentation. Critique the "A" section, and list what needs to be documented to make this a well-written progress note.*

_____

_____

_____

Practice Exercise 9 ➤ *You are on your last clinical affiliation at Happy Rehabilitation Center, where they use the SOAP format for documentation. Your patient is Jim, who has quadriplegia as a result of a spinal cord injury from a snowmobile accident. When he tries to sit, he faints because blood pools in his paralyzed legs, causing his blood pressure to drop (orthostatic hypotension). You have been working on a tilt-table treatment plan to overcome the orthostatic hypotension and to accomplish the anticipated goal of ability to tolerate the upright position for 30 minutes. The functional outcome is for Jim to be able to sit for 2 hours. It is Friday afternoon, and you are writing your weekly progress notes.*

Interpret the subjective and objective data in the A section of this incomplete note. Write in black ink.

1-20-06 Dx: Orthostatic hypotension 2° SCI C7.
　　PT Dx: Unable to tolerate upright sitting.

_____

S: Pt. continues to c/o dizziness when he attempts sitting.

O: Pt. has had 3 sessions on the tilt table to develop tolerance for upright sitting. First session BP dropped from 130/80 mm Hg to 90/50 mm Hg p̄ 10 min at 40° elevation. Today BP dropped from 130/80 mm Hg ā Tx to 100/60 mm Hg p̄ 15 min on tilt table at 50°. BP 125/75 mm Hg 5 min p̄ pt. returned to supine position.

A:

_____

_____

_____

_____

_____

_____

_____

_____

_____

_____

_____

_____

Practice Exercise 10 ➤ *You are on your second clinical affiliation at Mary Hospital and have been working with Sally, who burned her Ⓛ hip. You give her whirlpool treatments daily so the moving water will débride (i.e., clean out) the wound, and you use sterile technique to change the dressing. The goal is to promote healing of the wound so she will be able to sit properly and begin walking. You are writing your progress note after today's treatment session. Write the interpretation of the data portion of this incomplete note. Use black ink.*

11-2-06 PT Dx: Open wound due to 2nd-degree burn on Ⓛ gluteus medius, not able to sit with even wt.-bearing.

_____

Pt. reports itching around edge of wound. Pt. sat in whirlpool 100°F, 20 min, for wound débridement and to increase circulation for healing, sterile technique dressing change. No eschar, edges pink, 1 tsp drainage, clear, odorless. Diameter Ⓡ outer edge to Ⓛ outer edge: 4 cm today compared with 4-3/4 cm 10-31-06. Pt. sat in whirlpool with even weight-bearing on pelvis and taking support from arms on edge of whirlpool.

_____

_____

_____

_____

_____

_____

Practice Exercise 11 ➤ *Write the assessment of the data portion of this note.*

Dx: Subacromial bursitis Ⓡ shoulder.
PT Dx: Pain c/o, ROM deficit in all shoulder motions, and strength deficit in anterior and middle deltoid limiting ability to load luggage into trunk of taxi and work as a taxi driver.

_____

Expected Functional Outcome: Able to consistently load luggage into the trunk of the taxi with 0–3/10 pain rating in 10 days.

Anticipated Goals:

Pain rating reduced from 8/10 to 5/10 with shoulder movements for lifting and carrying objects in 5 days.

Consistent use of proper body mechanics using legs and minimizing shoulder motion for lifting, reaching, and carrying in 5 days.

AROM of all movements of the shoulder will increase by 50% of the AROM measured in the initial examination for lifting, reaching, and carrying in 5 days.

Subjective and objective information from your treatment session.

4-17-06

Pt. reported he was able to lift a passenger's briefcase today with no pain, guessed the briefcase weighed about 15 lb; rated his pain with shoulder flexion 6/10 before ultrasound and 4/10 after the ultrasound treatment. Pt. has not missed any appointments. This is the 4th visit. Direct US/subacromial bursa/sitting with shoulder extended/forearm resting on pillow/1 w/cm²/8 min/to increase circulation and decrease inflammation. Pt. correctly followed home exercise instructions for AAROM "wand" exercises for Ⓡ shoulder using a cane (see copy in chart). AROM Ⓡ shoulder flexion 0°–120° (0°–80° initial exam). Initiated body mechanics training for reaching into trunk of car, needed frequent verbal cues to keep arms close to body and weight shift with legs. Consistently demonstrated proper form for squatting and lifting, no verbal cueing needed (occ cues needed last visit for keeping head and shoulders up). Able to lift 30 lb from floor 5X (20 lb 5X last visit).

a. What would you write next in the interpretation of the data section?

b. Are the subjective and objective data recorded correctly?

c. Are the goals written correctly?

_____

_____

_____

_____

_____

_____

_____

_____

Practice Exercise 12 ➤ *Write the interpretation of the data section of this note:*

Dx: 4 weeks status post-surgery for herniated disc C4–C5.
PT Dx: ROM deficit in all cervical motions limiting ability to look around and over shoulders for safe driving.

Expected Functional Outcome: Able to return to safely driving in 2 months

Anticipated Goals:

AROM cervical rotation Ⓑ will improve 0°–45° to be able to see objects at shoulder level in 2 weeks.

Independent in performing HEP of cervical AROM exercises to be able to look over shoulders in 1 week.

S: Pt. reports having difficulty with "chin tuck exercises" at home, notices she can see more items on the wall in the garage when she tries to look over her shoulder.

O: Pt. has been seen 3 times. Passive manual stretching, all cervical motions, 30-sec hold, 5 reps, supine, to increase ROM. Pt. gave correct demonstration of all exercises in HEP (see copy in chart) but needed correction and cueing to pull occiput toward ceiling with "chin tuck" exercises. Quality of the exercise improved after 10 reps. Cervical AROM Ⓑ rotation 0°–30° before stretching, 0°–35° after stretching (0°–20° initially).

A:

_____

_____

_____

_____

Practice Exercise 13 ➤   *Write the interpretation of the data portion of this note:*

Dx: Ⓛ lower extremity bone cancer with above-knee amputation.
PT Dx: Ⓛ hip flexion/extension ROM deficit, L hip abductor strength deficit limiting ability to walk safely with prosthesis.

Expected Functional Outcome: Independent ambulation in home and community with prosthesis and appropriate ambulation aid in 1 month.

Anticipated Goals:

Hip flexion/extension PROM 0°–110°, hip hyperextension 0°–10°. Ⓛ hip abductor strength increase to lift 10 lb, 3 sets of 10 reps in 1 month. Ambulation with cane on carpet, grass, steps in 2 weeks.

Pt. states he is able to lie prone with one thin pillow under abdomen instead of two pillows for 1 hour. Missed yesterday's session because of the flu. This is pt.'s 5th session. HP/Ⓛ iliopsoas/20 min/to increase elasticity to prepare for stretching. Hip flexion PROM 15°–110° before HP, 10°–110° after HP. Contract-relax active stretching/ Ⓛ hip flexors/5xprone/to gain hip extension ROM. PROM hip flexion 5°–110° after stretching (20°–110° initial exam). Required frequent reminders to breathe while performing 10 reps active extension exercises, prone over one pillow. Exercise performed with effort, movements not smooth. Required occ verbal cueing to maintain Ⓛ leg in midline while performing Ⓛ hip abduction strengthening exercises, side-lying, using 4-lb cuff weight (up from 3-lb last visit), 3 sets of 10 reps, exerting effort last 3 reps and tending to hold breath. Provided written instructions (see copy in chart) and 4-lb cuff weight for this exercise to be continued at home. Gait training on grass with quad cane on Ⓡ (walker initial exam) requiring contact guard assist for safety with uncertain balance due to slight hip-flexed posture, uneven strides with shorter stance time on Ⓛ.

a.   Write the interpretation of the data information next.

b. Are the subjective and objective data written correctly?

c. Are the goals written correctly?

_____

_____

_____

_____

_____

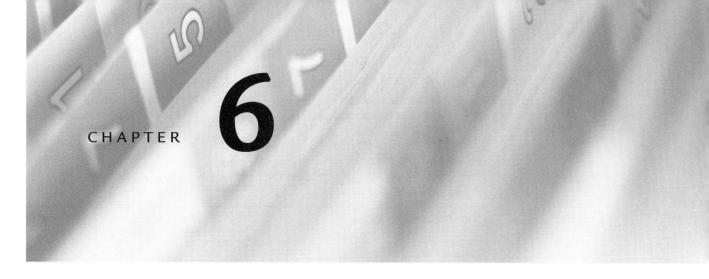

CHAPTER **6**

What Is the Plan and Why It Is Important

LEARNING OBJECTIVES

After studying this chapter, the student will be able to:

☐ Compare and contrast the plan content in the PT's evaluation with the plan content in the PTA's progress note.

☐ Discuss how the plan section incorporates the PT–PTA team approach to patient care.

☐ Incorporate the plan into the rest of the SOAP note or progress note.

INTRODUCTION

The "*P*" stands for *plan*. This information describes what will happen next. The PT's treatment plan is outlined in this section of the evaluation report. In the progress note, the PTA describes what he or she may need to do before and during the next treatment session.

The previous chapters have shown how the examination/evaluation report and progress note tell a story about the patient's physical therapy medical care. First, the patient's thoughts or contribution to the information is presented. Then, the objective facts are gathered and documented. Next, the information is summed up and given meaning. Finally, a plan is outlined telling the reader what interventions are proposed for the patient. This information is contained in the P section of the SOAP-organized note, the E section of the DEP model, and the second P section of the PSPG outline.

TREATMENT PLAN CONTENT

The content in the plan section is more detailed in the PT's evaluation report than the plan content in the progress notes the PTA completes. The APTA's *Guidelines for Physical Therapy Documentation*[1] states that treatment plans "shall be related to goals and expected functional outcomes, should include the frequency and duration to achieve the stated goals."

Plan Content in the Evaluation Report

The PT outlines the treatment plan designed to accomplish the anticipated goals and expected functional outcomes. The plan is documented in the plan section of the initial evaluation. The treatment is directed toward the physical therapy diagnosis and includes two parts: (1) physical therapy activities or interventions that treat the impairments contributing to the patient's functional limitations, and (2) training in the functional tasks described in the goals and outcomes. The PT's plan will include treatment objectives. Written the same way as goals, objectives contain action words (verbs), are measurable, and have a time frame. They document the rationale for each activity or intervention listed in the plan. Figure 6–1 provides three examples of documentation of intervention plans.

INTERVENTION PLAN #1

Dx: ⓡ hip trochanteric bursitis.
PT Dx: Hip abductor muscle weakness and discomfort limiting tolerance for walking and stair climbing required at work.
Expected Functional Outcome: To be able to walk from car in parking lot to office and to climb two flights of stairs without using a railing in 4 weeks for return to work.
Anticipated Goals:
1. To be able to walk equivalent of two blocks with minimal hip abductor limp and 3/10 pain rating in 3 weeks.
2. To be able to climb one flight of stairs using railing and with 3/10 pain rating in 3 weeks.
3. To be able to increase hip abductor muscle strength to 5/5 in 4 weeks.
Intervention:
1. Ultrasound to ⓡ trochanteric bursa, moderate heating effect, to increase circulation to decrease inflammation and discomfort.
2. Exercises, including home program, for hip abductor muscles to strengthen to grade 5/5.
3. Home program of structured, progressive walking and stair climbing activities to increase tolerance to the activities without aggravating the bursitis.
US and exercise 3X/week for 2 weeks, then 2X/week for 2 weeks with emphasis on self-management and monitoring of home programs and discontinuation of US. Pt. has appointment with physician in one month. Rehab potential is good.

INTERVENTION PLAN #2

Dx: Fractures of ⓛ olecranon process and ⓛ hip.
PT Dx: Immobility required to allow healing causing patient to be dependent in ADLs, transfers, and ambulation so is unable to return to home.
Expected Functional Outcome: At discharge time, patient will be able to transfer and ambulate with support for return to home.
Short-term Functional Outcomes:
1. To be able to transfer from bed <--> chair <--> toilet with SBA in 2 weeks.
2. To ambulate with platform walker for support on ⓛ from bed to bathroom, and 200 ft to be able to ambulate required distances in the home with SBA in 2 weeks.
3. To be able to ascend one step using walker and SBA to enter home in 2 weeks.
Intervention Plan:
1. Exercises to strengthen all extremities to aid transfers and ambulation. Exercise plan to include home program.
2. Training and practice for transfers from all types of surfaces as required in the home.
3. Gait training with platform walker on level tiled and carpeted surfaces and one step as required in the home.
4. Home assessment visit to clarify needs for transfer and gait training planning.
5. Educate patient and family on hip protection and safety precautions for safe functioning in the home.
Pt. to be treated bid for 2 weeks with discharge to home with support and continued physical therapy through home health agency. Rehab potential good.

INTERVENTION PLAN #3

Dx: 4 weeks post fractures of ⓛ olecranon process and hip with healing in process.
PT Dx: Limited ROM and strength in ⓛ elbow and hip causing patient to be confined to ADLs within her home and requiring SBA.
Expected Functional Outcome: Discharge plan is for patient to be able to transfer and ambulate independently in her home environment, and to join family for summer activities in motor home on lake.
Short-term Functional Outcomes:
1. To ambulate independently using single-end cane within the home in 3 weeks.
2. To ascend and descend stairs using single-end cane and the railing independently in 2 weeks.
3. To walk to the end of the dock using single-end cane and SBA to sit and fish in 3 weeks.
4. To climb steps into motor home using single-end cane and SBA in 3 weeks.
5. To perform home exercise program independently and accurately in 1 week.
Intervention Plan:
1. Home program of exercises to increase ROM and strength of ⓛ elbow and hip in preparation for ambulation with cane and independent ADLs.
2. Transfer and ambulation training with progression of assistive devices appropriate for safe change from platform walker to goal of single-end cane.
3. Ambulation training on grass and dock using assistive device.
4. Stair climbing training with assistive device and railing in home and into motor home.
Home health physical therapy 3X/week for 2 weeks and decrease to 2X/week for 1 week. Rehab potential is good.

Figure 6–1   Three examples of documentation of intervention plans.

As the patient's status changes and goals are met, only the PT may modify or change the treatment plan. These changes are documented in the interim evaluations. The PTA may **not** modify the treatment plan without consulting the PT. Discharge evaluations contain the plan for any follow-up or further treatment that may be required. When goals, functional outcomes, and treatment objectives are written correctly, the PTA can easily follow them to plan each treatment session and measure treatment effectiveness related to the patient's progress toward meeting the goals. (See Chapter 5 for more information.)

Plan Content in the Progress Note

The plan content in the PTA's progress note contains brief statements about the following:

1. What will be done in the next session to enable the patient to progress toward meeting the goals in the intervention plan
2. When the patient's next session is scheduled
3. What PT consultation or involvement is needed or when the next supervisory visit will be made
4. Any equipment or information that needs to be ordered or prepared before the next treatment session
5. The number of treatment sessions the patient has remaining before being discharged
6. Whether consultation with another health-care provider is needed, such as the primary care physician, OT, SLP, or nutritionist
7. Anything that the patient or caregiver may need to do prior to the next treatment session, such as purchasing shoes with greater support and stability or removing physical obstacles from the home

These statements typically contain **verbs** in the future tense. The verbs describe what will happen between now and the next treatment session or what will happen at the next session.

A comment about something specific the PTA wants to be sure to do at the next session goes in the plan section. This written comment serves as a self-reminder for the PTA (e.g., "Will update written home exercise instructions next visit," or "Will check skin over lateral malleolus this p.m. after patient has worn new AFO 6 hours"). It is also a way to inform another therapist who may be treating the patient at their next session of what should be accomplished.

When commenting elsewhere in the note about concerns, suggestions, or something that must be brought to the PT's attention, a statement is written in the plan section to indicate that the PT will be consulted or contacted (e.g., "Will consult PT about referring the patient to social services"). This ensures follow-through, quality continuum of care, and PT–PTA communication. When the progress note is written by the PTA, the inclusion of such a statement in the plan section provides evidence of PT–PTA teamwork and collaboration. When the situation does not require consultation or immediate communication with the PT, the PTA can demonstrate PT–PTA teamwork by referring to the PT's goals or plan in the evaluation (e.g., "Will ambulate patient on grass and curbs this p.m. per PT's goal in initial eval"). The PT–PTA teamwork can also be addressed in the "A" section of the SOAP note by stating that the patient is progressing towards the goals established in the PT evaluation.

When the progress note is the method for keeping track of the number of treatment sessions the patient is receiving, the number of sessions to be scheduled is reported in the plan section. The objective data may state, "Pt. has been seen for physical therapy 3X." The plan portion of the note may read, "Pt. to receive 3 more treatment sessions," "Pt. has 2 more approved visits to be scheduled," or "Pt. will return on 2-16-00, 2-23-00, and anticipate discharge on 3-1-00."

Examples of PTA Plan Documentation

Additional examples of plan content statements likely to be read in a PTA's progress notes include the following:

- "Will increase weights in PRE strengthening exercises next session."
- "Will discuss with PT patient's noncompliance with exercise program."
- "Will consult with PT about adding ultrasound to treatment plan."
- "Will notify PT that patient is ready for discharge evaluation."
- "PT will see patient next session for reassessment."

- "Will ambulate patient on stairs this p.m."
- "Will order standard walker to be available for treatment session on 8-4-00."
- "Will have blueprints for constructing a standing table ready for home visit on 9-11-00."
- "Pt.'s spouse will remove all throw rugs from the home to make the environment safe."
- "Pt. will discuss side effects of the medication with PCP at a later appt. today."

SUMMARY   The plan component of physical therapy documentation addresses what will happen during subsequent treatment sessions or in the future in general. The evaluations contain a treatment plan and objectives designed by the PT to accomplish anticipated goals and expected functional outcomes. The PTA carries out the treatment plan designed by the PT, with notations to contact the PT when the plan needs to be changed or modified. The PTA designs activities to help the patient progress within the guidelines described in the plan.

For the plan content in the progress notes, the PTA documents what is planned for the patient at the next session(s), telling the reader generally how the patient will make progress toward the goals. The plan section may also include (1) a reminder to do something more specific, (2) statements of intent to consult with the PT regarding any concerns or suggestions that were mentioned elsewhere in the progress note, and (3) the number of treatment sessions yet to be completed. A statement in the plan section that mentions communication with the PT reinforces and demonstrates the PT–PTA team approach to patient care.

REFERENCES   1. American Physical Therapy Association. (2002). Guidelines for physical therapy documentation. In *Guide to physical therapist practice*. Alexandria, VA: APTA.

Review Exercises

1. Discuss what the reader will find in the **plan** section of the PT's evaluation.

2. Describe the PTA's role in **designing** the intervention plan.

3. Describe the **content** of the plan section of a progress note.

4. Explain how the plan section of the progress note can **support** the PT–PTA approach to patient care.

5. Describe the **difference** between an anticipated outcome or goal and what should be listed in the plan section of a progress note.

PRACTICE EXERCISES

Practice Exercise 1 ➤ *The progress note in Figure 4–4 of Chapter 4 Part 5-30-06 is incomplete. Finish the note by writing the plan section, stating what you will do next. Use black ink, and sign the note with your legal signature and your title (SPTA).*

_____

_____

_____

_____

Practice Exercise 2 ➤ *Write "S" next to the subjective data statements, "O" next to the objective data statements, "A" next to the assessment data statements, and "P" next to the plan data statements.*

_____ 1. Pt. c/o pain with prolonged sitting.

_____ 2. Decubitus on sacrum measures 3 cm from Ⓛ outer edge to Ⓡ outer edge.

_____ 3. Pt. ambulates with ataxic gait, 10 ft max. assist of 2° to prevent fall.

_____ 4. Pt.'s Ⓡ knee flexion PROM increased from 30°–90° and he will see orthopedic surgeon tomorrow.

_____ 5. Ambulates c̄ standard walker, PWB Ⓛ, bed to bathroom (20 ft), tiled surface, min. assist 1X for balance, verbal cueing for gait pattern.

_____ 6. Pt. states he is fearful of crutch walking.

_____ 7. Pt. continues to have limited ROM in Ⓛ shoulder and remains unable to put on his shirt or winter coat without help following exercises today.

_____ 8. c/o itching in scar Ⓡ knee.

_____ 9. Pt. transferred from supine to sit c̄ min. assist and 3 reps today without any pain.

_____ 10. AROM is limited in elbow flexion by 10° today.

_____ 11. AROM WNL bil. LEs.

_____ 12. Pt. demonstrated adequate knee flexion during initial swing c̄ verbal cueing p̄ hamstring exercises.

_____ 13. Pt. remains dependent in bed mobility and was unable to perform a transfer from bed to chair with max. assist.

_____ 14. Pt. reported his pain level is decreasing with exercise and he will see the doctor tomorrow.

_____ 15. Pt. had increased strength in Ⓛ shoulder flexion from 3/5 to 4/5 from last week. Pt. would like to talk to the social worker and he was given the phone number.

_____ 16. Pt. shoulder range is improving and has increased another 20° since last week. Will discuss possible d/c with PT after next visit.

_____ 17. Pt. pivot transfers, NWB Ⓡ , bed ↔ w/c, max. assist 2X for strength, balance, NWB cueing.

_____ 18. Pt. rates Ⓛ knee pain 5/10 when going up stairs.

_____ 19. LUE circumference at 3 cm superior to olecranon process is 12 cm.

_____ 20. BP 125/80 mm Hg, pulse 78 BPM, regular, strong following exercise.

Practice Exercise 3 ➤   *From Figure 4–4 of Chapter 4, finish the plan section of the 11-12-06 note.*

1. _____

_____

_____

2. _____

_____

_____

Practice Exercise 4 ➤   *From Figure 4–6 of Chapter 4, complete the plan section. Two examples follow.*

1. The patient will be referred to OT for evaluation of fine motor skills. SV with PT will be on 5-5-06.

2. Pt. has met all goals outlined in initial plan of care and PT will be notified to complete reevaluation by 7-7-06.

_____

_____

Practice Exercise 5 ➤   *The following are treatment scenarios in which you are the PTA working on functional activities with your patients. Paint a picture of each patient's functioning as if being recorded in the subjective, objective, assessment, and plan sections of your progress note. It is not difficult to paint a picture of the patient's functioning. Mentally reproduce the treatment session, and write the plan at the end of your note.*

1. You instructed Mrs. Smith, who had severely sprained her right ankle, in crutch walking using a non–weight-bearing gait. Her ankle has been casted, and she is not allowed to bear weight on the right for 3 days. You fitted her with axillary crutches and taught her how to walk 100 ft on tiled and carpeted level surfaces; how to sit down and get up from bed, chair, and toilet; how to climb a flight of stairs with the railing on the right going up; how to manage curbs and two steps without using a railing; and how to get in and out of her car. Mrs. Smith safely ambulated and required only verbal cueing from you to climb the stairs. You gave her written crutch-walking instructions. Mrs. Smith stated that she is concerned because her sister had an allergic reaction to the pain medication that the doctor prescribed to her. She also said that there are two steps into her living room at

home. The PT's anticipated outcomes for this patient are to be able to ambulate independently in her home and at work following the doctor's prescribed weight-bearing restrictions. She will be seen again by the PT in 3 days when her weight-bearing restrictions will change.

P: _____

_____

_____

_____

_____

2. You supervised Jack while practicing his circuit of job-simulation activities using correct body mechanics for 20 minutes, 15 repetitions. Jack has had back surgery (laminectomy L4,5) and is preparing to return to work as a bricklayer. You observed that he consistently maintained his correct lumbar curve when squatting to lift bricks and shifting weight to spread the mortar. He did need body mechanics reminders when he lifted the wheelbarrow handles and while wheeling the wheelbarrow, especially for turns. He tended to bend from the waist to reach the handles and to twist his trunk when turning the wheelbarrow. Jack complained of increased back pain after pushing the wheelbarrow 25 ft with 35 lb of weight in it, but he stated that he forgot to take his pain medication until 5 minutes before the treatment session today. The PT's anticipated goals for this patient are to return to work as a bricklayer, which involves full ROM of back and trunk, ability to lift 50 lb, and push a wheelbarrow weighing 75 lb at least 50 ft.

P: _____

_____

_____

_____

_____

3. You taught Sally, a patient with paraplegia from a spinal cord injury, how to transfer from her wheelchair to the toilet by using a sliding board. Sally stated that she really did not see the point of learning this activity because she wished she had died in the accident that paralyzed her. She required constant instructions and cueing regarding safety precautions, and you needed to help push her across the board. The first two times that you attempted it, you felt as though you did most of the work. The third time she tried, she was able to slide herself from the chair to the toilet with only a little boost from you. However, when going from the toilet to the chair, it felt as though you and Sally exerted equal effort. You decided that you should talk to the social worker at the rehabilitation hospital about Sally's comment and inform your supervising PT. The PT's anticipated goals for this patient are to be able to complete all activities of daily living as independently as possible.

(hint: max. assist means the therapist does most of the work; mod. assist means the therapist and patient exert about equal effort; min. assist means the patient does most of the work)

P: _____

_____

_____

_____

_____

4. You provided gait training for Mr. Olson to learn to ambulate with a wide-base quad cane in his left hand. He had a stroke and has right upper and lower extremity weakness. You walked with him from his bed into the bathroom, to the bedroom window, out into the hall area in front of the door, and back to his wheelchair next to the bed. He walked this circuit five times, with a 2-minute rest in the wheelchair between each trip. You needed to hold his gait belt and to help him shift his weight to his right leg. He stumbled three times, but he was able to recover his balance without your help. During the fourth and fifth trips, he was able to shift his weight to the right appropriately without your help. Prior to treatment, the nurse informed you that Mr. Olson was started on an antacid medication last night and that he has an appointment for an MRI later this afternoon (you were planning on seeing the patient again today but will now only be able to see him once).

P: _____

_____

_____

_____

Practice Exercise 6 ▶ _Decide whether the following statement is an anticipated goal for a patient or whether the statement should be included in the P section of the SOAP note. Place a "G" next to the statements that are goals for the patient and a "P" next to the statements that should be in the P section of the SOAP note._

1. _____ Pt. will be instructed in independent donning and doffing of AFO at next session.

2. _____ Pt. will walk independently with WBQC on uneven surfaces up to 30 ft in 2 min.

3. _____ Pt.'s mother will call the PCP to ask about supplemental feedings.

4. _____ Pt. will be seen 1X/wk at home by PTA to work on independent amb. skills.

5. _____ Pt. will be able to reach overhead with Ⓑ UEs to comb hair and wash face, independently.

6. _____ Pt. will be seen at B.S. to work on independent bed mobility skills 2X/day by PTA.

7. _____ Pt. will be independent in bed mobility skills including rolling, moving up/down in bed, and moving from lying down to sitting in 2 days.

8. _____ PTA will discuss adding use of the whirlpool to the pt.'s HEP with PT.

9. _____ Pt. will be discharged by PT after 3 more visits.

10. _____ Pt. will receive TENS 3X/wk to decrease pain as per PT's plan of care.

11. _____ Pt. will report a decrease in pain of 8/10 to 4/10 on a descending pain scale following exercise sessions by the end of the week.

12. _____ Pt. will be instructed in home use of TENS unit by PTA at next treatment session.

13. _____ Pt. will be discharged from inpatient PT care and transferred to home health-care facility on Friday.

14. _____ PTA will contact PCP to find out about pt.'s WB status and report it to the PT.

15. _____ Next treatment session will be a joint visit with the OT.

CHAPTER 7

Putting the Pieces of the Puzzle Together

LEARNING OBJECTIVES	**SUMMARY**
INTRODUCTION	**REFERENCES**
REVIEW OF THE SOAP NOTE	**REVIEW EXERCISES**
SUBJECTIVE	**PRACTICE EXERCISES**
OBJECTIVE	
ASSESSMENT	
PLAN	

LEARNING OBJECTIVES

After studying this chapter, the student will be able to:

☐ Compare and contrast all parts of the SOAP note, including the subjective, objective, assessment, and plan sections.

☐ Select relevant subjective, objective, assessment, and plan information to document the patient's physical therapy diagnosis and treatment.

☐ Organize subjective, objective, assessment, and plan information for easy reading and understanding.

INTRODUCTION

In the preceding six chapters, the reader has reviewed the important information about the development of appropriate documentation and the parts that should be included in documentation, specifically a SOAP note format. The reader should now have a basic idea about the type of information to include in each of the four sections of a SOAP note, be able to identify information that is not appropriate, and be able to provide information that will make the treatment session reproducible for another therapist who may assume responsibility for the patient's care. As with any new skill, it will take the new therapist some time to be able to organize data in a SOAP note format, maintain organization of the overall note, and remember to put into the note the information that will ensure reimbursement and continued care. The therapist can refer to the APTA's *Guide to Physical Therapist Practice*, for further clarification.[1]

In addition, it is necessary for the PTA to complete a thorough review of the patient's chart, especially the section that includes the PT's evaluation of the patient. The PT should also have provided short- and long-term goals for the patient's plan of care. If the PTA was not present at the evaluation, this review of the patient's chart is a critical piece of the puzzle to provide appropriate care within the scope of practice for the PTA. It is also important that the PTA discuss any questions or concerns with the supervising PT to ensure that the plan of care developed by the PT is followed correctly by the PTA.

As previously reviewed, it is essential that any information related to the patient's care and treatment be appropriately documented in the SOAP note by the treating PTA. The PTA must address the short- and long-term goals set by the PT and make any necessary referrals for the patient's care. All of this information must be communicated to the supervising PT on a regular basis (this varies within facilities), and it is also the PTA's responsibility to ensure that the required supervisory visits are completed per the guidelines of the state in which the PTA practices.

REVIEW OF THE SOAP NOTE

Subjective

The *"S"* section contains the information that the patient or family member **tells** the therapist. Remember, subjective information must be given to you by the patient, a family member, or another interested party. The information you are given that you place in the medical record must be relevant to the patient's care and should not include any other type of information such as personal statements, information regarding another family member that is not relevant to the patient's care, or any other inappropriate comment (i.e., "patient reported her husband was drunk last night," "patient's husband states she will not fix his meals," "patient's friend stated that the patient went to the movies with another man, who was not her husband").

For this section of the SOAP note, it is vital that the PTA address any changes in the patient's pain level, level of function, poor responses to the previous interventions, or any new changes in the patient's condition. Common mistakes to avoid when writing subjective information:

- Not providing a comparison for pain level changes
- Providing information not related to the patient's care
- Providing information that would violate the Health Insurance Portability and Accountability Act (HIPAA) guidelines
- Correcting any mistakes made in the note

Please see the following example of subjective information:

S: written incorrectly

- The patient stated that his pain level today was an 8.
- The patient watched football last night and was not happy with the outcome.
- The patient's neighbor wanted to know what was wrong with her friend.
- The patient's pain level was 6/10 today.

S: written correctly

- The patient reported that his pain level was an 8/10 today.
- The patient was able to sit up for over 1 hour while watching TV last night.
- The patient's neighbor asked for information regarding the patient, and she was instructed to discuss this with the patient.
- Because the pain level was 8/10, the PTA needs to draw a single line through the 6/10 and put his or her initials and date above the mistake.

Objective

The *"O"* section of the SOAP note contains the objective data; that is, data that can be **reproduced** or **confirmed** by another professional with the same training as the person gathering the objective information. It must include measurable or reproducible tests and observations. Therefore, information reported to or by the PTA must meet these guidelines. This section provides the signs of the patient's pathology and describes how it has influenced the patient's function. Some examples include measurable range of motion, measurable strength, number of repetitions or sets in an exercise pattern, or the distance the patient can ambulate.

In the objective section, the PTA is responsible for ensuring that the initial measurements provided in the PT evaluation are improving and that the patient is not losing strength, function, or range of motion. The PTA is responsible for measuring strength, measuring functional change, and measuring changes in the range of motion during every treatment session to ensure that the patient is progressing within the plan of care and that the PT is given this information. It is important that any measurable information is included in this section. Common mistakes to avoid when writing objective information:

- Not providing a comparison with the evaluation measurement and the current treatment measurement

- Not providing measurable goals for length or type of surface when ambulating
- Not providing the amount of support necessary during the treatment session (contact guard, etc.)
- Not providing the type of assistive device used by the patient

Please see the following example of objective information:

O: written incorrectly

- The patient ambulated 50 feet today.
- The patient was able to transfer from the bed to the wheelchair today.
- The patient was able to complete knee extension exercises with a 5-lb weight.

O: written correctly

- The patient ambulated 50 feet using a FWW and standby assist 2X today on an even surface.
- The patient was able to transfer from the bed to the wheelchair by using a stand pivot procedure and contact guard assist 3X before he experienced fatigue.
- The patient was able to complete right knee extension exercises to 180° in a sitting position using a 5-lb weight, independently. The patient completed 10 repetitions and 3 sets without fatigue.

Assessment   The *"A"* stands for *assessment*. In this section of the SOAP note, the PT or PTA **summarizes** the S and O information and answers the question, "What does it mean?" In the assessment section, the PT interprets, makes a clinical judgment, and sets functional outcomes and goals based on the information in the subjective and objective sections. Again, the assessment section must include the short- and long-term goals. Short-term goals can be addressed by the PTA, whereas the PT should address the long-term goals.

In the assessment section, the PTA has the additional responsibility of ensuring that the short- and long-term goals are being met and the patient is making progress within the prescribed plan of care. This section is often confusing for PTAs, and many PTAs tend to put the objective information in this section by mistake. This section should address the patient's progress within the plan of care, suggest changes within the plan of care, and address any of the short- or long-term goal completions that might occur. Common mistakes to avoid when writing assessment information:

- Putting objective information in this section
- Changing the plan of care
- Changing the short- or long-term goals

Please see the following example of assessment information:

A: written incorrectly

- The patient completed all her short-term goals and new ones were added.
- The patient has completed all his goals and will be discharged tomorrow.
- The patient did not tolerate the treatment session so the plan of care was changed.

A: written correctly

- The patient was able to complete all of her short-term goals without fatigue today, and the PTA will communicate with the PT to change the plan of care and develop new short-term goals.
- The patient has completed all the goals set within the initial plan of care, and the PTA will discuss a possible discharge date with the PT today.
- The patient did not tolerate the treatment session today and became very fatigued following one repetition of knee extension with a 5-lb weight. This is a decrease in strength from the last session. The PTA will discuss this change with the PT and follow the new plan of care that will be developed.

Plan   The *"P"* stands for *plan*. In this section of the SOAP note, the treating therapist should include information about any **referrals** necessary for additional medical treatments, **when**

the next session will be, **how** many sessions there are until discharge, how many sessions there are until a supervisory session will occur, and **recommendations** for any equipment or home services before or upon discharge. This section should never include the anticipated goals for the patient's plan of care.

In this section, the PTA includes the number of treatment sessions left or being done per week, addresses a possible discharge date, makes referrals for other services as needed, addresses the time period for the next PT supervisory visit, and makes any other recommendations for equipment, etc. This information is also communicated to the supervising PT to ensure the plan of care is being followed. Common mistakes to avoid when writing "P" information:

- Not stating the number of treatment sessions left
- Not providing referrals as necessary
- Not addressing equipment needs
- Not setting up the supervisory visit with the PT
- Not signing the note correctly

Please see the following example of plan information:
P: written incorrectly or in a confusing manner

- The patient will be seen again.
- The patient is having fine motor problems.
- The patient needs a wheelchair.
- The PT will see the patient soon.

P: written correctly

- The patient has six more treatments before a reevaluation needs to be completed for insurance purposes. He continues to be seen 2X/week.
- The patient will be referred to the occupational therapist because of problems with dressing and shaving.
- The patient will need a manual wheelchair for discharge next week. Will communicate with the PT regarding type of wheelchair and date of discharge.
- The PT will make a supervisory visit on 1-20-07.

SUMMARY　As can be seen, the SOAP note format divides the patient treatment information into four specific sections, thereby providing an organized report of the patient's treatment and progress. This type of reporting provides the student or new therapist with the means to determine and report what happened during the treatment session, provides a means for another therapist to replicate the next session, maintains progress within the plan of care, and moves the patient toward discharge and return to the individual's highest functional level.

REFERENCES　1. American Physical Therapy Association. (2003). Guidelines for physical therapy documentation. In *Guide to physical therapist practice* (2nd ed.). Alexandria, VA: APTA.

2. American Physical Therapy Association. (2003). Documentation for physical therapist patient/client management. In *Guide to physical therapist practice* (2nd ed.). Alexandria, VA: APTA.

Review Exercises

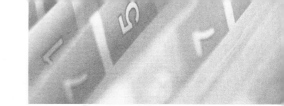

1. **Describe** the importance of each section of the SOAP note. Give an example of each one.

2. What is the **purpose** of the goals in the assessment section?

3. Can the PTA discharge a patient? Why or why not?

4. List **three** activities that could be included in the **objective** section of the SOAP note.

5. List one **appropriate** statement for the subjective section and one **inappropriate** statement for the subjective section.

Practice Exercise 1 ➤ *Write "S" next to statements that describe the subjective portions of a note, "O" next to the statements that fit the objective data category, "A" next to the statements that fit the assessment data category, "P" next to the statements that fit the plan data category, and "N/A" next to an inappropriate comment.*

_____ 1. Pt. was able to complete an additional five repetitions of exercise program.

_____ 2. Will refer pt. to OT for evaluation of hand function.

_____ 3. Will set up supervisory visit with PT by 3/15/06.

_____ 4. Pt. ambulated 50 feet with FWW and SBA.

_____ 5. Pt. stated she went to the store last night.

_____ 6. Pt. referred to social worker for preparation for discharge on 3/15/06.

_____ 7. Pt. stated she had pain relief of 8/10 for several hours after last treatment session.

_____ 8. Pt. able to ambulate 150 ft independently.

_____ 9. Pt. will be able to independently ascend four steps with one hand rail and rec. gait by next visit.

_____ 10. Will increase weights for shld. abd from 5-lb to 20-lb with reps the same.

_____ 11. Will recommend SLP referral before next visit and communicate to PT.

_____ 12. Pt. PROM in SLR measured at 165°.

_____ 13. Pt.'s husband stated she had a fever last night after session was completed.

_____ 14. Pt. has increased pain following stretching and strengthening program today.

_____ 15. Pt. performed knee flexion to 98° on CPM for two 60 minute sessions without increased pain/swelling.

_____ 16. Pt. states the session went well last visit with no increase in pain and slight increase in swelling.

_____ 17. Will continue seeing pt. for therapy session 3X/week.

_____ 18. Will increase pt. ambulation from mat exercises, independently, 100 ft with crutches.

Practice Exercise 2 ➤ *In the following note, organize the information in a SOAP note format and circle reproducible statements.*

Increase wts. in hip extension from 2-lb to 3-lb by the end of the session; reviewed home ex. program with pt., and pt. was able to complete an appropriate and safe-return demo; pt. states that pain has decreased from 9/10 to 7/10 with strengthening exercises in shld. horiz.

abd with yellow theraband and 10 reps/3 set done once a day at home; will refer patient to OT for eval of wrist range and strength; refer pt. to neurologist for eval of arm tingling and pain; pt. PROM in shld. flex. measured 90° before exercise session and 110° following ex. with no complaint of increased pain; Pam is a 40-year-old patient with tenderness in the bicipital groove during active shld. flex. and horiz. abd; will speak with PT about next supervisory visit on 4/5/00; pt. questions home exercise of shld. horiz. abd because it hurts to do it and it did not hurt during the last treatment session; pt's overall UE strength was 4/5 following the treatment session today.

_____

_____

_____

_____

_____

_____

_____

_____

_____

_____

_____

_____

_____

_____

_____

Practice Exercise 3 ▶   *In the following note, organize the information in a SOAP note format, use approved abbreviations, and circle reproducible statements.*

This is the first patient you are seeing this morning. Anthony is a 65-year-old male who underwent thoracic surgery to remove a cancerous section of his left upper lobe yesterday. Your supervising PT completed the evaluation last night. The patient completed shoulder ROM exercise on the left side today, shoulder flexion to 45° and shoulder abduction to 45° doing 10 repetitions each. The patient is sitting with the head of the bed elevated to 45° when you enter his hospital room. The patient stated that he knew the pain would be bad, but he didn't realize it would hurt as much as it does. He rated his pain as a 9/10 on a verbal rating scale. You demonstrated to him, again, how to produce the most effective cough by bracing a pillow over his chest, and he then accurately demonstrated it back to you. You will see this patient for a second visit later this afternoon. You informed the patient that when he is lying down, he should keep the head of the bed at 30° with his hips and knees slightly flexed to reduce pressure on his chest and decrease his pain. He has a posterior-lateral incision. The patient stated that he tried to cough last night holding a pillow over his chest like the PT showed him, but he does not know if he is doing it right. He completed 3 sets of 10 reps of ankle pumps with each side and did 5 SAQ with each leg. You decide that you should ask the PT when the patient will be allowed to begin to get out of bed and start ambulating. The patient was able to cough bracing with the pillow 3X during the treatment session. The PT goals are to increase total lung volume by teaching the patient to have an effective cough, pain management, prevent DVTs, and regain normal active and passive ROM in left shoulder.

_____

_____

_____

_____

_____

_____

_____

_____

_____

_____

_____

_____

Practice Exercise 4 ▶   *Place a check mark next to the statements that are written correctly and identify, by rewriting the statement, which portion is incorrect.*

1. _____ Increase Ⓛ ankle ROM to 25° of plantarflexion.

   _____

2. _____ Will discuss pt.'s noncompliance with HEP with PT.

   _____

3. _____ US to Ⓡ gluteal area.

   _____

4. _____ Pt. able to amb. 30 ft in 2 min today, 4 min yesterday.

   _____

5. _____ Pt. demonstrated decrease in Ⓛ LE strength.

   _____

6. _____ Pt. complained of hip pain.

_____

7. _____ Pt. will perform UE PNF patterns diagonally.

_____

8. _____ Pt. stated he was able to ambulate to the end of his driveway and pick up his newspaper this a.m.

_____

9. _____ NWB Ⓡ UE.

_____

10. _____ Ⓡ shld. not assessed.

_____

11. _____ Diameter of wound Ⓡ outer edge to Ⓛ outer edge: 5.5 cm at eval. last Tuesday, 4.0 cm today.

_____

12. _____ LE strength N at knee and hip.

_____

13. _____ Pt. is left-handed.

_____

14. _____ ROM G in Ⓑ UEs.

_____

15. _____ Pt. will receive US to Ⓡ upper trapezius at 1.0 W/cm^2 for 7 min.

_____

PART THREE

How Do SOAP Notes Ensure Good Patient Care?

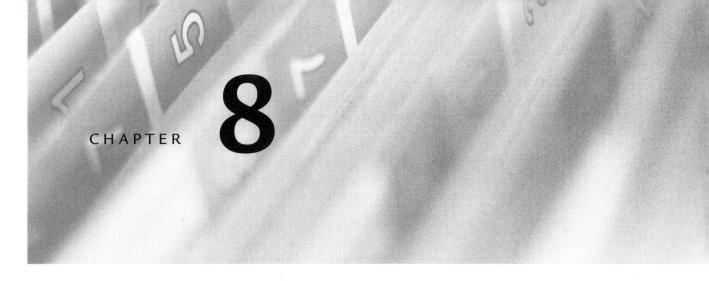

CHAPTER 8

How Does Documentation Relate to Patient Issues?

LEARNING OBJECTIVES

After studying this chapter, the student will be able to:

☐ Compare and contrast the differences between functional outcomes and limitations.

☐ Assess specific types of communications related to patient treatment, and determine the scope of practice responsibilities related to the PT's and PTA's treatments.

☐ Discuss general requirements related to patient confidentiality and relate these requirements to HIPAA practices.

☐ Identify the time frame and be able to develop a report for any incident causing injury to a patient during a treatment session or while the patient is under the care of the PTA.

☐ Differentiate between medical and educational therapy services.

INTRODUCTION

In addition to recording the physical therapy care of the patient, the PT and PTA share other document responsibilities. All clinical facilities have documentation procedures for recording telephone communications, HIPAA practices, incident reports, patient noncompliance, and patient refusal of care. In addition, any care provided by a PT or PTA must be medically or educationally appropriate and must determine whether therapy is necessary or only providing maintenance of patient skills. With all documentation, one of the most important considerations is patient confidentiality.

TYPES OF OUTCOMES

There are several types of outcomes related to patient care in the therapy setting. It is always important to be able to determine whether the treatment necessary meets an educational goal or a medical one. The PT and PTA can use functional levels and limitations to help determine some of these goals.

Functional Outcomes

These outcomes are directly related to the patient's prior level of function (PLOF), the medical and physical therapy diagnoses, the patient's functional limitations, the assessment of the referred problem, the development of a treatment plan, and input from the patient.

Patient's Limitations

When dealing with referrals for physical therapy, the PT and PTA must be cognizant of the patient's limitations. Such limitations may or may not be directly related to the physical therapy diagnosis. The physical therapist will decide whether the limitation the patient is experiencing can be improved with the development of the physical therapy plan of care. If not, the limitation could interfere with or decrease the success of the physical therapy. This limitation may or may not affect the patient's functional level. Any limitation must be evaluated to determine if the limitation will aid in returning the patient to the previous level of function.

Medical Necessity

Medical necessity determines the type and frequency of physical therapy intervention. The treatment must be "reasonable and necessary" to receive reimbursement. The medical condition that resulted in the referral may not be the sole reason for physical therapy. For example, a patient who has experienced a CVA does not automatically have a medical reason for physical therapy. Just because the patient suffered a stroke does not mean he needs physical therapy. The fact that the patient now has left-sided paresis and can no longer ambulate independently may be one reason for the referral. It is important to document the actual reasons for the physical therapy referral and why physical therapy will benefit the patient and will return the patient to a higher functional level.

Educational Necessity

Physical therapy provided in a school setting can be very different from that provided in a medical setting. For the student to receive physical therapy in the school setting, he or she must meet certain criteria. The student may qualify for physical therapy in the school system when the student cannot move about in the school environment, cannot ambulate independently, or has balance and coordination problems.

For example, the PT receives a referral for physical therapy for a child with Down Syndrome. The child can ambulate independently, moves throughout the school environment without help, but cannot climb the ladder to go down the slide. The parent is demanding that her child receive physical therapy for this reason and because he has Down syndrome. Following the PT's evaluation, it is determined that the child is 5 years old, can walk independently, can run awkwardly, and can ascend and descend stairs with the help of two hand rails and by marking time. Because the child can ambulate and move about the school environment independently, he does not qualify for physical therapy in the school setting. Down Syndrome cannot be the reason he receives therapy. Because he has difficulties on the playground, the PT might refer him for an adaptive physical education evaluation instead.

Maintenance Therapy

One determinant against physical therapy relates to the necessity for those services. For the adult patient who does not show any progress, who has met the goals and objectives of therapy, or who has received the amount of therapy allowed by the paying entity, therapy is now considered a maintenance service. If the patient is not showing any improvement in function or has completed all the therapy sessions allotted by the insurance company, such as Medicare or Medicaid, the physical therapy is no longer "reasonable and necessary." Therefore, physical therapy is no longer appropriate for the patient, and the patient will be discharged from services.

However, for the pediatric patient, maintenance therapy is not such a deterrent for services. Through numerous state and federal agencies' support, pediatric patients may receive physical therapy services from the time of birth until they are 21 years old. From birth to 3 years old, these patients may be enrolled in an early intervention program. From 3 to 21 years old, they may receive services through the school system. Even if the patient does not show improvement in function, physical services can still be provided if the PT determines that they are needed. The only requirements relate to the student's ability to have access and to move safely in the school environment.

For instructions and regulations related to physical therapy care and treatment, the reader can go to the following Center for Medicare and Medicaid's (CMS) Web page: www.cms. hhs.gov/providerupdate. The quarterly report, *The CMS Quarterly Provider Update*, includes all changes to Medicare instructions that affect medical providers, provides a single source for national Medicare provider information, and gives medical providers advance notice on upcoming instructions and regulations.

PATIENT CONFIDENTIALITY

All medical records and information regarding the patient's condition and treatment are confidential. Only those health-care professionals providing **direct** care to the patient have access to this information. Any individual not providing direct care to the patient must be authorized by the patient to receive information about his or her medical care and condition. This is an ethical principle commonly called the *rule of confidentiality.*

General Requirements

The patient provides authorization for sharing his or her medical information by signing a release-of-information form for each health-care organization or by naming each person to whom the information can be released. Figure 8–1 is an example of a release-of-information form.

The PTA may not provide information about the patient to anyone without first knowing whether the person is authorized to receive the information. This includes the patient's spouse or any other relative, neighbor, or friend. Once authorization is obtained, then the facility's procedure for releasing information is followed.

The patient's medical record is kept in a secure location, such as behind the nursing station counter or in a secure office with limited access to prevent unauthorized persons from reading it. The PTA respects this rule of confidentiality by returning the patient's medical record to its proper location or by passing it on to another authorized person. The record must never be left lying unattended on a counter or desk. Also, never leave documents with a patient's confidential information unattended at a copy machine. If you must make photocopies of any part of a patient's medical chart, remain with the documents at all times and make sure to remove all of the documents from the copy machine. Any discussion about the patient's condition must occur in private areas and only with the patient, caregivers, and those authorized to receive the information.

Any researcher who wants to gather information from the medical record must also have the patient's permission. The researcher cannot publish or reveal the patient's name or any other descriptions that would identify the patient.

The Patient's Rights

Although the health-care facility is the legal owner of the medical record, the patient has the legal right to know what is in it. The patient must follow the facility's procedure to access his or her record. Usually the procedure simply involves asking the patient to sign a request form. The PTA needs to be knowledgeable about the facility's procedure.

HIPAA Requirements

The Health Insurance Portability and Accountability Act of 1996 (HIPAA), or *Standards for Privacy of Individually Identifiable Health Information,* which, after undergoing several revisions, has been mandated by the federal government to protect the individual and all information related to the person's health care. These standards were revised by the Department of Health and Human Services (HHS) on April 14, 2003. These new standards gave the patient more control over their medical records and more protection regarding who had access to them.

HIPAA provides provisions regarding electronic transactions and covers all health plans, health-care providers, and those individuals or facilities that conduct administrative transactions (such as billing). Reasonable safeguards must be initiated to protect the patient that include the following steps:

- While discussing a patient's condition with family members or other health-care providers, move the conversation to a private conference room or office.

Release of Information Form

Patient Name_____ DOB _____
Address: _____ Social Security # _____

I authorize and request XXX Medical Rehabilitation Center to release records maintained while I was a XXX patient, disclosing information as specified below. This form may be utilized for several parties to eliminate duplicate paperwork.

PURPOSE OF REQUEST:

__X__ Insurance Reimbursement   _____ Worker's Compensation
__X__ Subsequent Treatment/Intervention on behalf of patient   _____ Damage or claim eval. by attorney
_____ Other (Specify) _____

INFORMATION TO BE RELEASED:

__X__ Eval Reports   __X__ Discharge Reports
__X__ Progress Notes   __X__ Physician Order(s)
__X__ Plan of Care   __X__ Other (Specify)_____

By placing my initials in the appropriate space, I specifically authorize XXX to include in the records released, information relating to or mentioning the following, if any:

_____ Psychological conditions   _____ Drug or alcohol abuse

RELEASE:

*1. Release to: *Physician*   *2. Release to: *Insurance Company*
   Name: Name:
   Address: Address:

*3. Release to: *Employer*   *4. Release to: *QRC or Disability Case Manager*
   Name: Name:
   Address: Address:

5. Release to: *Attorney Law Firm*   6. Release to: *Patient*
   Name: Name:
   Address: Address:

7. Release to: 8. Release to:
   Name: Name:
   Address: Address:

*When a therapist requests courtesy copies, the above parties signified by an asterisk (*) will automatically receive copies of medical records.

REVOCATION

I understand that I may revoke this authorization at any time. If I do not expressly revoke this authorization sooner, it will automatically expire 1 year from the date of this authorization; or under the following conditions:

   a.) authorization may extend beyond one year if this is a worker's compensation case.

   b.) other (specify) _____

COPIES

A photocopy of this authorization X may _____ may not be accepted by you in place of the original.

SIGNATURE

_____   _____
Signature of patient or person   Date
authorized to sign for the patient

If signed by someone other than the patient, state how authorized _____

REFUSAL

I do not wish to authorize release of information to the following individual party(ies)

_____
Name of party or parties

_____   _____
Signature   *Date*

Figure 8–1   Example of a release-of-information form.

- Avoid using the patient's name or even a description of the patient in hallways and elevators, and post signs to remind employees to protect the patient's confidentiality.
- Isolate and lock filing cabinets or records rooms.
- Provide additional security, like computer passwords, to secure personal information.

In addition, HIPAA provides several provisions to further protect patients:

- Provides for patient access to medical records with the right to correct errors within 30 days of a written request. Patients may be charged for the cost of copying and postage.
- Provides for patient information about how their medical records will be kept and their rights will be protected in regards to the medical care they receive and the individuals who have legal access to that information.
- Provides for patient information about the method of disbursement of their medical information and an acknowledgement that this information was shared with the patient's written permission.
- Protects patients from the marketing of any information related to their medical care without written authorization while allowing patients access to disease-management information.
- Informs patients that state regulations can overrule HIPAA in circumstances such as the reporting of an infectious disease outbreak to public health authorities.
- Provides patients' the right to file a complaint with the Office of Civil Rights (OCR) when they feel their rights regarding their medical information have not been honored. Complaints can be filed by calling 1-866-627-7748 or accessing the following Web page: www.hhs.gov/ocr/hipaa.

Employers and employees must also follow guidelines related to sharing medical information:

- Written policies and procedures must be in place to provide protection regarding patient information related to any medical care from those individuals that might have access to such information.
- Employees have been trained in privacy policies and procedures, and disciplinary procedures are in place if those procedures are violated.
- Disclosure policies related to emergency situations, public health needs, judicial proceedings, and certain law enforcement activities have been relayed to employees.
- Employees have been trained to disclose any information that may affect national defense or security.

Third-Party Payer Guidelines

In addition to Medicare and Medicaid, third-party payers, such as health maintenance organizations (HMOs), private insurers, and Champus or Tri-Care for military families, provide reimbursement for physical therapy services. Most of these companies follow the reimbursement policy of the CMS. If Medicare or Medicaid will not pay for a service, chances are that any other type of insurance will also refuse to pay for that service. The most important component of reimbursement is being attentive to the policies and procedures of that insurance company. It is also helpful to provide detailed written requests that address the need for the treatment and the expected goals and outcomes.

Types of Communication

The PTA may participate in three common types of telephone conversations requiring documentation in accordance with the facility's policies and procedures:

Telephone Referrals

1. Taking verbal referrals for physical therapy treatment from another health-care provider
2. Receiving information about the patient from the patient or a representative of the patient
3. Receiving inquiries about the patient's medical condition or about the physical therapy treatment from interested persons, provided that the patient has signed a release of information form enabling the sharing of such information

Other Referrals for Physical Therapy

Referrals for physical therapy services may be telephoned to the department by other health-care providers or their staff. Telephone orders for physical therapy services may be made by a physician, a nurse, or a receptionist acting under the physician's direction. One PT may call and refer a patient to another PT with expertise in the treatment of a patient's particular condition. Another health-care provider, such as an occupational or speech therapist, may telephone a referral because physical therapy is the more appropriate medical treatment for the condition of his or her patient.

When receiving a referral over the telephone, the PTA should follow the facility's procedure for documenting the call. Carry a pen and notebook in your pocket at all times to allow quick note taking when answering the telephone. Take notes to gather the information to document later. Use the facility's form for recording telephone referrals. A copy or a similar form with the information from the call is sent to the referring provider for signature. This signature proves that the conversation and referral did take place. Typically the documentation requirements for a telephone referral include the following:

- Date of the call
- Name of the person phoning in the referral and the person's relationship with the patient
- Name of the primary care physician
- Name of the PTA answering the telephone and receiving the verbal referral
- Details of the referral and accompanying information regarding the patient
- Comment regarding plans to send written verification of the telephone referral to the referring party
- Comment indicating that the referral will be brought to the attention of the PT

Information From or About the Patient

The PTA may answer the telephone when a patient or family member calls to report a change in the patient's condition or ability to keep a therapy appointment. If the call is about a change in the patient's condition, the PTA may need to refer the caller to the PT or the patient's physician. If it is an emergency situation, the caller is advised to transport the patient to the emergency room or to call 911. Documentation about this call may include:

- Date and time of the call
- Name of the person calling and their relationship to the patient
- Name of the PTA taking the call
- A summary of the conversation, including the response of the PTA
- A comment regarding the apparent emotional state of the caller (tone of voice, disposition, orientation)

Request for Information About a Patient

Often persons other than those providing direct patient care have an interest in the patient's condition and treatment and may telephone to inquire about the patient's progress. Attorneys, insurance representatives, parents of children less than 18 years of age, other relatives, friends, and neighbors are examples of persons who might call the physical therapy department. For example, a patient who was injured while working may have lawyers, a rehabilitation manager, an insurance representative, and an employer, all of whom may want to know about the patient's medical care. When the PTA answers the telephone and the caller asks about a patient's condition, the PTA must follow the rules of confidentiality.

PROTECTING THE PATIENT

Along with keeping patient confidentiality, the PT and PTA have a responsibility to protect the patient in other ways. These ways include, but are not limited to, informed consent, proper tool use, proper use and filing of an incident report, and legal responsibilities related to the treating therapist.

Informed Consent

Informed consent is defined as "a legal condition whereby a person can be said to have given consent based upon an appreciation and understanding of the facts and implications of an action." The individual needs to be in possession of all of his faculties, such as not being mentally retarded or mentally ill and without an impairment of judgment at the time of consenting. Impairments include illness, intoxication, drunkenness, using drugs, insufficient sleep, and other health problems" (www.ama-assn.org/ama/pub/category/4608.html).

Consequently, informed consent means more than giving permission to treat. In addition, all aspects of the treatment plan, including the purposes, procedures, expected results, and any possible risks or side effects of treatment, must be explained to the patient and/or significant others. If possible, it is usually best to have the patient participate in designing the plan.

The patient or the patient's representative then decides whether to accept the treatment plan or refuse it. This policy and procedure ensures that the patient is not being coerced into any course of action. This consent may be informal and verbal or formal and written. When the patient gives a verbal consent, the PT documents the consent in the initial evaluation. In many medical facilities, a formal informed consent form or document must be signed before treatment is initiated. When a patient is receiving physical therapy, the PT designs the treatment plan and reviews the plan with the patient. Thus, the appropriate person to obtain the informed consent signature is the PT, not the PTA. Once signed, this form is placed in the medical record.

An informed consent document should contain the following:[1]

1. A description of the physical therapy diagnosis and the proposed treatment plan written in language that the patient or the representative of the patient can understand
2. Name and qualifications of the responsible PT and other physical therapy personnel likely to be providing the care
3. Any risks of or precautions to the treatment procedures that the patient should consider before deciding to agree to or refuse the treatment
4. An explanation of any alternative treatments that would be appropriate, including risks or precautions that need to be considered if the alternative treatment is used
5. The expected benefits of the proposed treatment plan and the expected outcomes if the physical therapy problem is not treated
6. Responsibilities of the patient or representative of the patient in the treatment plan
7. Answers to patient's questions

Proper Tool Use

Using Black Ink

Use of black ink is a common guideline but is subject to change. Black ink traditionally had been used because it photocopied more clearly than other ink colors. However, photocopy technology has progressed so that other ink colors now copy clearly and print black. Now, some lawyers are having legal documents signed in blue ink to distinguish the original from the copy. Other colors such as green, mauve, or taupe may copy well but are inappropriate for a medical record. The PTA should follow the facility's procedure.

Falsifying Information

In every case, it should be difficult for someone to change or alter the written note. To ensure that no opportunities exist for changing or falsifying the information, follow these guidelines:

1. Do not use erasable pens.
2. Do not erase errors.
3. Draw a line through the mistake, and date and initial directly above the error (e.g., patient ambulated with ~~crutches~~ ML/3-4-06 standard walker).
4. Do not leave empty lines or spaces at the end of a sentence, a section, or a completed therapy note. Empty spaces provide the opportunity for someone to add or change information, thus falsifying the record. Draw a horizontal line through empty spaces (see Fig. 8–2).

Timeliness

Complete the documentation as soon as possible after seeing the patient, while the information is fresh in your mind. A progress note written immediately after the patient treatment session is the most accurate note. However, it is more likely that the PTA may move from one patient to the next and treat a full day's schedule of patients before being able to document.

The patient will be seen 2X/wk for six weeks. Will contact PT for supervisory visit after six visits.

_____ Tom Therapist, LPTA

Figure 8–2 Example.

> **9-12-06** AM   **Dx:** Ⓛ hip fracture.
>   **PT Dx:** Dependent with pivot transfer.
> **S:** Patient states she performed a pivot transfer from the chair <—> bed with minimal help from daughter last night.
> **O:** 9-12-06 ss. After three trials, pt. stood & pivoted non–weight-bearing on left, chair <—> mat, WC <—> toilet, bed <—> WC with SBA for loss of balance recovery if needed. No loss of balance.
> **A:** Pt. ready for pivot transfer with SBA with nursing. Making good progress toward goal of independent transfers.
> **P:** Will notify PT & nursing. _____ Sally Student, SPTA/Mary Therapist, PT (Lic. #)
>
> **9-12-06 10:00** AM   Pts. vital signs were taken by LPN following breakfast and PT session. BP was 135/85, temp was 99°, resp. 15/minute and pulse 80 BPM.
>
> **9-12-06 10:00** AM   Blood work completed for pro time and potassium levels per physician order.

Figure 8—3   An example of a patient's note during one day.

Carry a small notebook to take notes while treating the patient so that each patient's progress note will be accurate and thorough.

Treatments that are provided twice a day may be documented by placing a.m. or p.m. after the date (12-4-00 a.m.) (12-4-00 p.m.). This allows another health-care provider, such as the OT, nurse, or speech pathologist, to document in the progress note section of the chart between the physical therapy a.m. and p.m. notes, thus illustrating the continuum of care throughout the day (refer to Fig. 8–3).

An addendum is made when information is added to a note that has already been written and signed. To add more information later, date the new entry and state "addendum to physical therapy note dated 6-21-06." Refer to Figure 8–4 as an example of a progress note that follows legal guidelines.

Incident Reports

An *incident* is anything that happens to a patient, employee, or visitor that is:

- Out of the ordinary
- Inconsistent with the facility's usual routine or treatment procedure
- An accident or a situation that could cause an accident

All medical facilities should have a policy and procedure for documenting incidents in an *incident report*. During the first or second day of internship or on a new job, the student or the newly employed PTA should read the facility's instructions for completing and filing an incident report.

Purpose of an Incident Report

The incident report is used for risk management and legal protection. Following the policy and procedure for reporting incidents protects everyone who uses the facility (i.e., all patients, employees, and visitors) from future incidents. The procedure describes a method for providing a prompt response to medical needs, identifying and eliminating problems, and gathering and preserving information that may be crucial in litigation. The report contains information that identifies dangerous situations that either caused or could cause an injury.

> **9-12-00** AM   **Dx:** Ⓛ hip fracture.
>   **PT Dx:** Dependent with pivot transfer.
> **S:** Patient states she pivoted chair <—> bed with minimal help from daughter last night. _____
> **O:** 9-12-00 ss. After three trials, pt. stood & pivoted non–weight-bearing on left, chair <—> mat, WC <—> toilet, bed <—> WC with SBA for loss of balance recovery if needed. No loss of balance. _____
> **A:** Pt. ready for pivot transfer with SBA with nursing. Making good progress toward goal of independent transfers. _____
> **P:** Will notify PT & nursing.
>
>   Sally Student, SPTA/Mary Therapist, PT (Lic. #)

Figure 8—4   An example of a progress note following legal guidelines.

Risk managers use this information to change the situation, thereby reducing the risk for injury. The incident report alerts the administration and the facility's lawyer and insurance company to the possibility of liability claims. It "memorializes important facts about an alleged incident that create a record for use in further investigation."[4]

Legal Responsibility When an Incident Occurs

Only the eyewitness fills out and signs the incident report. If more than one person witnessed the incident, one of the eyewitnesses completes the report but includes the names of the other witnesses. The person documenting the incident must follow the facility's procedure. The incident report is completed on a form unique to the facility. Most medical facilities use similar forms, which typically ask for the following information:

1. *Name and address of the person involved in the incident:* When the person involved is an employee or visitor, his or her home address is given. If the person is a patient, the patient's address, date of birth, gender, admission date, and status before the incident are provided. The patient's medical diagnosis and physical therapy diagnosis are recorded along with a brief summary of the care the patient has received.
2. *An objective, factual description of the incident:* The PTA completing an incident report does not express an opinion, blame anyone or anything, or make suggestions

---

PREDISPOSING CONDITIONS

Diagnosis: Fx (R) hip   hypertension

Mental Status (i.e., Oriented, Alert/Confused, etc.): -alert & oriented

List pertinent medications if applicable: Tylenol   lanoxin   tenex

Follow up measures to Incident:
MD & family notified, vital signs checked every 2 hours for 12 hours

Was a Medical Device Involved?   ☐ Yes   ☒ No   Manufacturer's Name and Address (if Available on Equipment or Packaging):

Type ——————— Model No. ———————
Serial No. ——————— Lot No. ———————

Incident Reported By: Joan Anderson ——————— Title: PTA

Date of Report: 11/21/00	Signature & Title of Person Preparing Report: Joan Anderson/PTA

Reviewed by DON: Virginia McDormel/Rn ———————   Reviewed by Administrator: Mike Bond ———————
            (Signature)   (Signature)

Date: 11/22/00 ———— Charted: ☒ Yes ☐ No   Date: 11/23/00 ————

Reviewed by Medical Director: Dr Steve Jones ——————— Date: 11/30/00 ———————
            (Signature or initials)

DO NOT WRITE BELOW THIS LINE-TO BE COMPLETED BY ADMINISTRATOR/DON

Vulnerable Adult Report Made?   ☐ Yes ☒ No

Incident Reported To (Circle as many of the following as applicable.):

Local Welfare Agency   Local Police Department   County Sheriff's Office   Office of Health Facility Complaints

Other (Explain) ———————

Date Report Called in (Within 5 Days): ———— Approximate Time: ———————— ☐ a.m. ☐ p.m.

Name of Person Spoken to: ———————— Reported By: ————————

Date Report Mailed: ———————— To Whom: ————————

incident.rep

Figure 8—5A An example of the front of a completed incident report.

```
┌──────────────────────────────────────────────────────────────────────────┐
│                          ABC HEALTH CENTER                                 │
│                          INCIDENT REPORT                                   │
├────────────────────────────────────────┬───────────────────────────────────┤
│ Resident/Visitor #1   Jane Doe          │ Resident/Visitor #2    n/a        │
├────────────────────────────────────────┼───────────────────────────────────┤
│ Address: 7700 Grand Ave.               │ Address:                          │
│          Duluth                         │                                   │
│                                         │                                   │
│ Phone #: 628-2341    DOB 1/17/17        │ Phone #:            DOB            │
├────────────────────────────────────────┼───────────────────────────────────┤
│ Date: 11/21/06   Time  2:30   am/pm     │ Location of Incident: P.T. Dept   │
└────────────────────────────────────────┴───────────────────────────────────┘
```

Description of Incident:
Pt was standing in parallel bars with PTA holding on with transfer belt, Pt performing ® L/E standing exercise, she became pale and dizzy, could not walk back to chair, was lowered to floor by PTA. Never lost consciousness, felt much better once reclined. With assist of RPT was lifted into w/c

Assessment: Describe injury (if any) in detail:
Skin tear on ® forearm when arm hit bar while lowering small 1.5X 2.0 open area with small amount of blood

Name/Title of All Witnesses:
Mary Smith/RPT
Joan Anderson/PTA

Safety Measures in Use:
Transfer Belt: __X__
Siderails: __does not__
Restraint: __use__ Type: _____

Intervention: None Required _____   At Facility __X__

Describe:
Vital signs checked and charted in nursing chart, skin tear was cleansed & protective covering in place. ROM to U/E & Ⓛ L/E WFL s̄ pain! ® L/E ROM within hip precaution limits s̄ pain

Resident #1

Hospitalized: Yes ___ No _X_	Date _n/a_ Time ___ am/pm	Hospital _n/a_
Physician Name: Harvey Jones	Notified by: Dana Olson/RN Date 11/21/06 Time 3:00 am/pm
Family Name: Robert Doe/son	Notified by: Dana Olson/RN Date 11/21/06 Time 3:15 am/pm

Resident #2 n/a

Hospitalized: Yes ___ No ___	Date ___ Time ___ am/pm	Hospital ___
Physician Name:	Notified by:	Date ___ Time ___ am/pm
Family Name:	Notified by:	Date ___ Time ___ am/pm

Figure 8–5B   An example of the back of a completed incident report. The names and situation are fictitious.

as to how the incident might have been prevented. The incident is to be described as the eyewitness saw it, not as someone else described it. No secondhand information is to be included in the report. The circumstances surrounding the incident, the condition of the affected person after the incident, and the course of action taken are described.

3. *Identification of all witnesses to the event:* The report includes addresses of the witnesses, if known, as well as identification of the equipment involved by model number and manufacturer.

Each facility has a time period within which the report should be submitted. This can vary from 24 hours to 3 days after the incident. Because the incident report is not considered part of the medical record, it is placed in a file separate from the patient's medical record. The PTA must document the incident in the patient's chart; however, the PTA does not mention that an incident report was completed. The report is a confidential, administrative document for use in case of litigation and for risk-management review and action. Box 8–1 summarizes the "do's and don'ts" of incident reporting.[2] Figure 8–5 is an illustration of a completed incident report. The names and the situation are fictitious.

> **Box 8–1   Summary of Do's and Don'ts of Incidence Reporting**
>
> 1. DO notify your PT.
> 2. DO know your facility policy and procedure for reporting an incident.
> 3. DO write legibly and use professional terminology.
> 4. DO include names and addresses of employees or visitors who know anything about the incident.
> 5. DO give the completed report to your supervising PT to route for the necessary signatures.
> 6. DON'T mention that you've filed an incident report in the patient's chart.
> 7. DON'T photocopy an incident report.
> 8. DON'T write anything in the report that implicates or blames anyone for the incident.
> 9. DON'T use incident reports for disciplinary actions.
> 10. DON'T use the report for complaining about co-workers or other employees.
> 11. DON'T talk about the incident with noninvolved personnel. Remember *CONFIDENTIALITY*.
> 12. DON'T acknowledge any incident or give any information until you've checked with your PT or a supervisor.
>
> Adapted from Documentation, In Clinical Pocket Manual. Nursing 88 Books. Springhouse Corporation, Springhouse, PA, 1988, pp. 135–136.

Patient Refusal of Treatment

As discussed in this section and in Chapter 2, after receiving information about all aspects of the treatment, the patient or a representative of the patient must consent to the treatment plan. The patient does have the right to disagree with the plan or to change his or her mind later and refuse treatment.

When a patient refuses treatment, there are several things the PTA can do:

1. Use active listening skills, interview, and talk with the patient to try to determine the reason for refusal. The patient may have a very good reason why it would not be appropriate to receive treatment at that time. For example, a gentleman in a nursing home refuses therapy without explaining why. After spending some time talking with him, he reveals that his dog had passed away the previous evening. This man is grieving his loss and would not be able to concentrate on his therapy activities.
2. If there does not seem to be a reason for the refusal, make sure the patient fully understands the purpose of the treatment and the expected outcomes if the problem is not treated.
3. If the patient continues to refuse, recognize the patient's right to refuse, document this in the patient's chart, and notify the PT.

Documenting Treatment Refusal

The PTA documents the patient's statement of refusal of treatment and the reason for refusal. The PTA describes his or her response and action taken. A statement about notifying the PT is included. The documentation may read as follows:

8-3-06

1:00 p.m.: Pt. refused treatment this p.m. After being encouraged to attend at a later time, pt. stated her sister was visiting from out of state and the only time she would be able to visit with her was this afternoon. She expected her soon and anticipated the visit would last all afternoon. Agreed to cancel treatment this p.m. and scheduled pt. for tomorrow a.m. Will notify PT.

—Bob Smith, LPTA

SUMMARY   The PT and PTA are responsible for documenting numerous events and tasks occurring during the course of a day. The PTA must know the facility's procedures for documenting various types of conversations, documenting necessity, maintaining the patient's confidentiality, providing the patient with informed consent, understanding incident reports, and documenting the patient's refusal of treatment. General descriptions of these common events and their procedures were discussed in this chapter.

REFERENCES   1. Scott, R. W. (1994). *Legal aspects of documenting patient care* (pp. 123–125, 183). Gaithersburg, MD: Aspen.
2. Hilton, D. (ed.). (1988). *Documentation: A clinical pocket manual* (p. 135). Springhouse, PA: Springhouse Pub. Corp.

Review Exercises

1. Explain the difference between **medical** and **educational** necessity.

2. List **three** requirements you can address to protect patient confidentiality.

3. What is an **incident report** and why is it important in patient care?

4. Who is responsible for **completing** an incident report and why is it not filed in the patient's medical record?

5. What is **HIPAA** and what do the initials represent?

6. Your patient's neighbor brought her to therapy today. She wants to know how her friend is doing and why she is receiving PT. What, if anything, can you tell her and why?

7. An attorney representing your patient in a lawsuit phones and wants an update on the patient's progress. What is the PTA's best response?

Practice Exercise 1 ➤ *From the following list of statements, identify the statements that the PT, PTA, or both might write in a SOAP note by marking them with a "PT," "PTA," or "B."*

1. _____ The patient stated their pain had decreased from 8/10 to 6/10 following treatment today.

2. _____ The patient has been discharged on 2-3-06 for noncompliance.

3. _____ PROM is WFL in the Ⓡ UE.

4. _____ The patient's wife stated that he did not sleep last night because of pain.

5. _____ The patient was able to ambulate with CGA for 100 ft using a FWW on linoleum.

6. _____ The next supervisory visit with the PT will be on 4-21-06.

7. _____ Will refer patient to OT services for an evaluation.

8. _____ Reevaluation will be done on the next visit on 9-8-06.

9. _____ Strength in the Ⓛ LE hip flexion is 3/5 with PROM/AROM WNL.

10. _____ Will review progress and plan of care in next department team meeting.

Practice Exercise 2 ➤ *Identify the statements that indicate medical necessity, educational necessity, or both by marking them with an "M," "E," or "B."*

1. _____ Pt. will increase strength from 3/5 to 4/5 in triceps by 3rd visit.

2. _____ Pt. will ambulate, within the school building, independently using a posterior walker.

3. _____ Pt. will transfer from wheelchair to desk, independently, with SBA.

4. _____ Pt. was shown the home program and successfully performed a return demo.

5. _____ Pt. stated that she could not lift the 5-lb weight in shoulder flexion and used less weight.

6. _____ Pt. will demonstrate a safe and independent transfer from the chair to a mat.

7. _____ Pt. will receive PT services 3X/week in the classroom and gym setting.

8. _____ Pt. has increased AROM in Ⓑ UE shoulder abduction.

Practice Exercise 3 ➤ *From the statements given, identify the statement that will maintain patient confidentiality under HIPAA guidelines by marking it with a "P". If the statement violates patient confidentiality, explain why and mark it with a "V". Explain why your answers protect or violate patient confidentiality.*

1. _____ Calling the patient by their first name to notify them you are ready for their treatment.

2. _____ Having all the patients sign in at the front desk.

_____

3. _____ Telling the friend what is wrong with her neighbor.

_____

4. _____ Telling the parent what progress their child has made during therapy.

_____

5. _____ Sending patient information to the referring doctor.

_____

6. _____ Receiving a pt. referral by telephone.

_____

7. _____ Letting the patient look at their chart.

_____

8. _____ Giving the pt. a diagnosis in the waiting room.

_____

9. _____ Allowing the SLP to review the therapy notes on your patient.

_____

10. _____ Reporting the patient's noncompliance in a team meeting.

_____

Practice Exercise 4 ➤ *Identify the statements given below that warrant an incident report by marking them with an "I."*

1. _____ The patient slipped through the gait belt but was caught by the therapist before falling.

2. _____ The patient fainted while sitting on the edge of the bed.

3. _____ The patient fell while ambulating in the hallway.

4. _____ The patient received a minor burn from the UV lamp.

5. _____ The patient felt dizzy and was moved to a chair while ambulating.

6. _____ The patient fell out of bed and was found on the floor.

7. _____ The patient fainted while on the commode.

8. _____ The patient left the facility AMA.

9. _____ The patient mentioned that she had stubbed her toe last night.

10. _____ The patient fell down the stairs while using crutches.

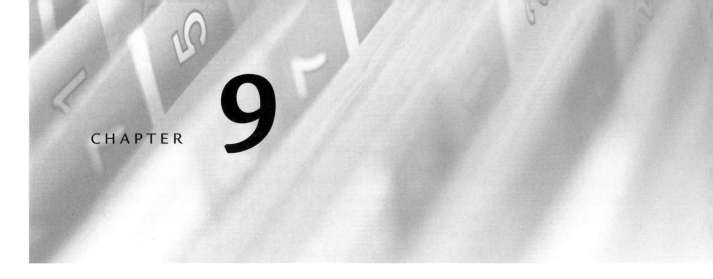

CHAPTER 9

Your Documentation Related to Legal and Ethical Issues

LEARNING OBJECTIVES

After studying this chapter, the student will be able to:

☐ Organize information to present documentation at state and federal court hearings.
☐ Review of professional liability and its importance in the legal setting.
☐ Definition of a deposition.
☐ Explanation of the responsibility of the PTA when testifying in a legal setting.
☐ Review of ethical standards of practice for the PTA.

INTRODUCTION

Part of a therapist's responsibility in documentation is to provide information when requested to appear in a civil, state, or federal court proceeding, on behalf of a patient or the medical facility for which they work. Any therapist that provides documentation can be subpoenaed (a formal written order to produce documentation or appear in court) to testify in a court proceeding for the prosecution or the defense. As seen in the example in Chapter 1, the PT and the PTA could be called for either side. It is imperative that the patient documentation be comprehensive and reproducible and can stand on its own in a court hearing. Generally, most medical records should be kept from 3–6 years. However, some medical facilities keep them for 7 years while others store them indefinitely. For liability purposes, it is important for the PTA to know how long these records should be kept according to state statutes and individual medical facility policy. General HIPAA guidelines require medical facilities to retain their patient records for 6 years. Following a patient's death, the record must be kept for 2 years. Hospitals must maintain their patient records for 5 years (http://www.hipaadvisory.com/regs/recordretention.htm). Records related to minors should be retained until the minor reaches legal age (dependent on the state) or the statute of limitation for that state.

PROFESSIONAL LIABILITY INSURANCE

As for the PT, the PTA must also maintain professional liability (malpractice) insurance to provide legal protection in case of litigation. This type of insurance is usually provided through the medical facility for which the therapist is employed. However, some facilities (e.g., small outpatient clinics, clinics in rural settings) do not provide this type of insurance, and the PT or PTA should have a personal insurance policy. Several companies offer such insurance, which can be reviewed at the following websites: www.hspo.com, Healthcare Providers Service Organization (HPSO), or https//secure.lockton-ins.com, the American Council of Healthcare Professionals. The annual fee for this type of insurance is from $100 to $200, depending on the company, the PTA's number of years in practice, whether the PTA is employed or self-employed, and whether the PTA practices in more than one medical facility.

Professional liability insurance should cover the employed, self-employed, or student therapist on and off the job. This type of coverage will protect the treating therapist if litigation occurs and will provide legal representation if the medical facility does not do so. Minimum coverage should include the following:

- Up to $1,000,000 each claim professional liability coverage
- Up to $3,000,000 aggregate professional liability coverage
- Occurrence-based coverage
- Defense cost payment
- Deposition representation
- Defendant expense benefit
- License protection
- 24-hour coverage

Additional coverage may include:

- Assault coverage
- Personal liability coverage
- Personal injury coverage
- First-aid expense
- Medical payments
- Damage to the property of others

LEGAL ISSUES

Testifying in Court

Most therapists are very apprehensive about the first time they have to testify in court. A summons to appear in court can be very intimidating, but if you have appropriately documented the care given to the patient and have performed within your scope of practice, you should have nothing to worry about. During the court proceedings, you will be called to testify and will be sworn to tell the truth when giving your account of the situation, as you remember it. One of the primary mistakes made when requested to testify in court is to provide **too** much information. Simply answer the questions that are presented to you in a clear and concise manner without elaboration. Also, be prepared to have your documented notes projected onto a screen for everyone to see and read. Penmanship and spelling do matter! Any documentation related to patient care must be included (see Box 9–1).

As therapists, we tend to want to help, and this can be a poor idea in any legal setting. The best rule of thumb is to answer "only" the question asked. It is important not to elaborate on any one question and to let your documentation speak for itself. Remember, you are there to protect your patient, defend the care that was provided, and prove that you treated the patient within your scope of practice and that you followed the recommendations of your supervising physical therapist.

In addition, you must tell the truth, the whole truth, or … well, you get the idea. You can support the truth best by having accurate, comprehensive, and understandable documentation. You may not be called to testify about a particular patient for months or even years after you

---

Box 9–1   Court Documentation

Any note completed on behalf of the patient and the care they have received can be entered into court as a document of record. The method of documentation does not matter. If the notes were handwritten, transcribed from a recorder, or placed on a computer, any and all forms must be produced when the individual receives a subpoena.

have treated them. It is important that you be able to read your documentation, because you will not be able to recall every detail about every patient that you have treated. If you have penmanship that even you cannot read, you could be placing your patient, your facility, or yourself in unnecessary jeopardy.

Depositions

A deposition, also know as examination before trial (EBT), is the act or fact of taking sworn (under oath) testimony from a witness outside of court. The deposition is written down by a court reporter for later use in court. It is a part of the discovery process whereby litigants obtain information from each other in preparation for trial (http://www.nolo.com/definition. cfm/term). Some jurisdictions recognize an affidavit, a written declaration made under oath before a notary public or other authorized officer (http://www.1stoplegal.com/forms/ affidavits.htm or wordnet.princeton.edu/perl/webwn) as a form of deposition.

Depositions are taken for the purpose of discovering the facts upon which a party's claim is based, such as obtaining financial information or discovering the substance of a witness's testimony prior to trial. The deposition may be used to discredit a witness if he changes his testimony or may be used to preserve the testimony of a witness who will be unable to appear at trial (www.brandeslaw.com/Legal_dictionary/legal.htm). In addition, some depositions may be taken by using a digital video deposition system whereby the individual may be deposed from a remote location, making travel and time away from work more cost-effective. This type of deposition is available 24/7, can be reviewed for changes, and becomes part of the permanent record.

For the PTA requested to attend a deposition, the lawyers will be present for both the prosecution and the defense, and both lawyers will be able to ask you questions. The PTA will be sworn in during this proceeding to ensure the accuracy of the responses. The main differences between a court hearing and a deposition are the environment in which the deposition is held and the fact that the PTA will be able to review the information and make changes before it is entered into court. Most depositions are held in a lawyer's office, a public building, conference room, etc. The proceeding will be taped and/or documented by a court reporter. Again, because this is a legal proceeding, it is important for the PTA to answer the questions asked and not elaborate by providing more detail than necessary. Answers should remain concise and to the point, and the PTA should expect his or her documentation to support the care given.

Statements

Sometimes a general statement will be requested of the PTA. This is not usually required in a court setting or in a deposition, nor is it under oath. This may be part of an information gathering process to determine whether a court hearing is necessary or whether an arbitration hearing might be possible.

In an arbitration hearing, the participants do testify under oath and all parties have agreed to the results of the arbitration decision. Because this is not a court hearing, substantial court costs are not incurred and issues are more quickly settled. However, again, the PTA must answer only the questions asked and not elaborate any further.

ETHICAL ISSUES

When giving any statements related to the care of a patient, you must determine whether the patient's rights and confidentiality are being protected by meeting HIPAA guidelines. Under the HIPAA guidelines, any medical information related to the patient's care can be used in a deposition or court hearing (refer to Chapter 8). However, any medical information is accessible to the patient with a written request. Patients have the right to have copies of their medical records, can request changes in those records, and can decide with whom those records can be shared. With the evolution of HIPAA in 1996, patient confidentiality requirements makes adherence to these guidelines paramount (refer to the following Web page for additional information on HIPPA requirements, www.cms.hhs.gov/ providerupdate).

In addition, the PTA is bound by professional ethics and conduct, as outlined in the ATPA's *Guide to Physical Therapist Practice*.[1,2] The APTA's code of ethics for PTAs is listed in Box 9–2. These documents also can be found at the APTA Web site: www.apta.org.

Box 9–2	APTA Standards of Ethical Conduct for the Physical Therapist Assistant

HOD 06-00-13-24
(Program 17) [Amended HOD 06-91-06-07; Initial HOD 06-82-04-08]

Preamble
This document of the American Physical Therapy Association sets forth standards for the ethical conduct of the physical therapist assistant. All physical therapist assistants are responsible for maintaining high standards of conduct while assisting physical therapists. The physical therapist assistant shall act in the best interest of the patient/client. These standards of conduct shall be binding on all physical therapist assistants.

Standard 1
A physical therapist assistant shall respect the rights and dignity of all individuals and shall provide compassionate care.

Standard 2
A physical therapist assistant shall act in a trustworthy manner towards patients/clients.

Standard 3
A physical therapist assistant shall provide selected physical therapy interventions only under the supervision and direction of a physical therapist.

Standard 4
A physical therapist assistant shall comply with laws and regulations governing physical therapy.

Standard 5
A physical therapist assistant shall achieve and maintain competence in the provision of selected physical therapy interventions.

Standard 6
A physical therapist assistant shall make judgments that are commensurate with their educational and legal qualifications as a physical therapist assistant.

Standard 7
A physical therapist assistant shall protect the public and the profession from unethical, incompetent, and illegal acts.

From the American Physical Therapy Association, Standards of Ethical Conduct for the Physical Therapist Assistant. Accessed March 13, 2007 from http://www.apta.org, with permission.

These guidelines for ethical conduct ensure that the PTA provides appropriate and ethical care to the patient by following the plan of care outlined by the supervising PT. It is imperative that the PTA communicate on a regular basis with the supervising PT to ensure that the plan of care remains appropriate and that the PTA continues to remain within the scope of practice as outlined in the state practice act. It is the responsibility of the PTA to ensure he or she has reviewed those regulations for every state in which he or she has a license to practice. By graduating from an accredited physical therapist assistant school, the PTA is further ensured of introduction to and follow through of such ethical conduct.

These standards are nationwide and should be followed despite the type of facility, the number of hours a PTA works, who the supervising PT might be, or the medical facility for which the PTA works. As for the PT, these standards of ethical conduct are in place to protect the patient, provide appropriate care, and maintain treatment under a plan of care developed and supervised by a licensed PT.

SUMMARY   This chapter provides the PTA with the necessity and importance of appropriate and comprehensive documentation in the care of any patient included in his or her caseload. The PTA must recognize the importance of this type of documentation, regardless of the format, in order to protect the patient, the treating PTA, the supervising PT, and the medical facility itself. The PTA must be held accountable for appropriate documentation that addresses the scope of practice in the state for which he or she has been licensed.

It is the responsibility of the PTA to provide treatment under the supervision of a licensed PT and to be able to defend the care given to any patient by following the plan of care outlined by the supervising PT. The PTA must also know and understand the standards of ethical conduct presented by the APTA to ensure appropriate and ethical patient care. By following these standards, the PTA can ensure that the care given will be appropriate and ethical even if the PTA receives conflicting information from the supervising PT. If the PTA remains within the scope of practice dictated by the state practice act for which he or she serves, the PTA can ensure that the patient will be protected and the care given will be accurate. As always, it is the PTA's responsibility to ensure the care he or she gives is appropriate for the patient's condition and within the PTA's scope of practice.

REFERENCES   1. American Physical Therapy Association. (2003). *Guidelines for physical therapist practice* (2nd ed.). Alexandria, VA: APTA.
2. American Physical Therapy Association. Standards of ethical conduct for the physical therapist assistant. Accessed March 31, 2007 from http://www.apta.org.

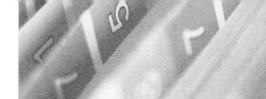

Review Exercises

1. Describe the **importance** of keeping legible and comprehensive SOAP notes of patient care.

2. **Why** would a PTA need to testify in a legal setting?

3. What are **two** differences between giving a deposition and testifying in a court of law?

4. How **long** should medical records be kept by the facility for which you work?

5. What is **HIPAA** and why is it so important?

6. Give **two** examples of how the PTA might **violate** HIPAA guidelines.

7. You have followed the plan of care outlined by your supervising PT to perform joint mobilization to a patient's right shoulder. You have performed Grade 4 joint mobilizations on the patient's shoulder causing a tear in the rotator cuff. Because you followed the plan of care outlined by the PT, **are you liable** for the injury? **Why or why not?**

8. In question 7, which standard of ethical conduct did you **violate**?

9. Following the treatment session, your patient has requested a copy of their medical records from your facility. Are you allowed to release a copy to the patient? **Why or why not?**

10. You are working with a patient and stretching the heel cords, following the plan of care outlined by the supervising PT. Suddenly, you feel the heel cord release and the patient cries out in pain. The back of the ankle suddenly starts to swell. You immediately put ice on the ankle, call the supervising PT to notify him of the injury, and recommend an x-ray of the ankle to determine the extent of the injury. You also complete an incident report to document what happened and the treatment given to the patient following the injury. The patient heals well with no further problems, the doctor reviews the x-rays and finds no bony injury, and the patient does not appear to have any further complaints. Two years later, the patient decides to sue your facility because of this injury, claiming he does not have full range of motion in the injured ankle. As the treating PTA, do you think this patient will be successful? **Why or why not?**

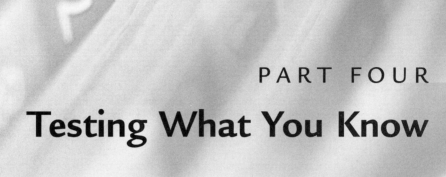

Testing What You Know

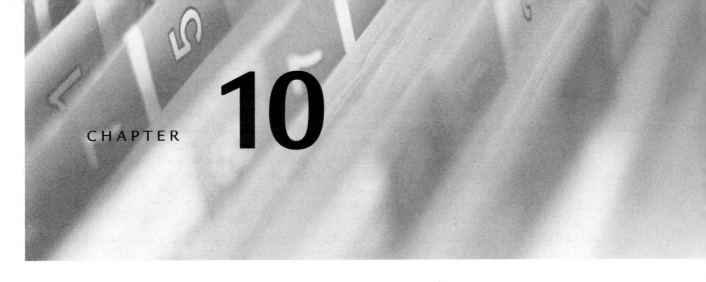

Do You Know Enough?

LEARNING OBJECTIVES

After studying this chapter, the student will be able to:

☐ Compare and contrast all parts of the SOAP note, including the subjective, objective, assessment, and plan sections.

☐ Select relevant subjective, objective, assessment, and plan information to document the patient's physical therapy diagnosis and treatment

☐ Organize subjective, objective, assessment, and plan information for easy reading and understanding

INTRODUCTION

As a student and a clinical practitioner, the documentation that you provide can mean the difference between payment for services rendered or denial of those services. Proper documentation is also important to help protect the patient, the medical facility for which you work, and ultimately, you. In addition, appropriate documentation ensures that the patient receives the correct care for the level of skill of the practitioner. The PTA is bound by the standards of ethical conduct to ensure that the patient is safe and that the PTA meets the scope of practice requirements for the state in which he or she is licensed.[1]

LICENSING EXAMINATION QUESTIONS

Questions on the national licensing exam related to SOAP notes are usually very generic and nonspecific. The questions asked will test the student's ability to think critically through a scenario, determine what types of comments and measurements should be included in each section, and demonstrate how to make the patient's next session reproducible by another therapist. If the student, as a practicing clinician, can meet those guidelines, he or she will have a firm grasp on the appropriate information to include in a SOAP note and the methods necessary to ensure the note can be followed by another therapist for continuity in the patient's care.

THE PTA'S RESPONSIBILITIES

As a student, you are required to produce appropriate documentation of patient care. This documentation should ensure that any other therapist providing care to this patient can follow the plan of care, progress the patient within the plan of care, and make recommendations for continued therapy, discharge, or referral to other services. The PTA remains responsible for the patient's care until the patient is discharged from therapy services by the supervising PT.[1] The PTA is also responsible for providing ethical and appropriate care that falls within their scope of practice of the state in which they are licensed. In this way, the patient receives appropriate and consistent care when receiving physical therapy services.

SUMMARY   As can be seen, the SOAP note format divides the patient's treatment information into four specific sections (subjective, objective, assessment, and plan), thereby providing an organized report of the patient's treatment and progress. This type of reporting provides the student or new therapist with the means to track and report what happens during the treatment session, provides a means for another therapist to replicate the next session, aids in the progression of the patient within the plan of care, and moves the patient toward discharge. Documentation also ensures that the patient is receiving quality care to help him or her recover to the highest functional level.

REFERENCES   1. American Physical Therapy Association. (2003). Guidelines for physical therapy documentation. In Guide to physical therapist practice (2nd ed., pp. 699–712). Alexandria, VA: APTA.

The following multiple-choice questions review all areas of a SOAP note and help prepare the reader for questions he or she might expect on the licensing examination and protect the therapist from litigation.

1. Identify the statement that would be placed in the **subjective** section of a SOAP note.

    a. AROM has increased to 90° in the (L) LE knee extension.

    b. The patient stated her pain is a 9/10 today.

    c. Harry was able to ambulate with CGA 50 ft using a quad cane on the right side.

    d. The patient demonstrated a correct home program following the session today.

2. Identify the statement that would be placed in the **objective** section of a SOAP note.

    a. Shoulder flexion measures 120°, an increase of 10° from the evaluation.

    b. The patient will be referred to OT for an evaluation.

    c. The patient increased ambulation from 50 ft to 100 ft during today's session.

    d. The patient stated she did not sleep well last night.

3. Identify the statement that would be placed in the **assessment** section of the SOAP note.

    a. The patient stated that her husband drank too much last night.

    b. The patient has completed the short-term goal of 10 reps and 3 sets of shld. flex.

    c. The patient will see the orthopedic surgeon next week.

    d. The patient was able to ambulate to his mailbox yesterday.

4. Identify the statement that would be placed in the **plan** section of the SOAP note.

    a. The patient has stopped taking her pain medication because it makes her sick.

    b. The patient demonstrated a proper home program today.

    c. The patient needs to return to the surgeon for a follow-up appointment.

    d. The patient's family wants her to come home.

5. Identify the **incorrect** statement that should **NOT** be in the subjective section of a SOAP note.

    a. The patient complained of increased pain (8/10 from 5/10) with hip abduction.

    b. The patient's mother states that he is difficult to listen to during her TV show.

    c. The patient stated that the swelling has decreased in the knee.

    d. The patient will make an appointment with the physician next week.

6. Identify the **incorrect** statement that should **NOT** be in the objective section of a SOAP note.

    a. The patient's (L) UE AROM has increased 15° since the last treatment session.

    b. The patient took her pain pill 30 minutes before the treatment session today.

    c. The patient has met the short-term goal of independent sitting.

    d. Active shld. flex. is 150°.

7. Identify the **incorrect** statement that should **NOT** be in the assessment section of a SOAP note.

    a. The patient states she was able to drive to the therapy session today.

    b. The patient completed 9/10 reps and 3 sets of her exercises.

    c. The patient complained that her husband is not helping around the house.

    d. The patient complained of increased swelling in her neck.

8. Identify the **incorrect** statement that should **NOT** be in the plan section of a SOAP note.

    a. The patient reported his pain was 9/10 when he arrived today for his therapy session.

    b. The patient c/o increased tightness in shld. ext. after yesterday's session.

    c. Will discuss the referral of pt. to SLP for evaluation in team meeting.

    d. Physical therapy will continue 2X/week with a reevaluation on 7-9-06.

9. Identify the statement that would be included in the **subjective** section of a SOAP note.

    a. The patient completed 3 reps of the exercise program.

    b. The patient stated his pain was 5/10 prior to exercising.

    c. The patient's mother stated they were going on a 3-month cruise.

    d. The patient reported he wanted to commit suicide.

10. Identify the statement that would be included in the **objective** section of a SOAP note.

    a. The patient completed 10 reps in 3 sets for hip flexion against max. resistance.

    b. The patient will be referred to OT for an evaluation.

    c. The patient will return for one more visit before the supervisory visit.

    d. The PT has increased the sessions for next week from 2X/week to 3X/week.

11. Identify the statement that would be included in the **assessment** section of a SOAP note.

    a. The patient stated that the exercises were too difficult and pain increased.

    b. The patient will see the orthopedic physician next week.

    c. The patient completed all of his short-term goals.

    d. The patient will be referred for a speech evaluation.

12. Identify the statement that would be included in the **plan** portion of the SOAP note.

    a. The patient requested that the spouse not be involved in the therapy session.

    b. The patient stated that they are able to complete all exercises and wants to increase them.

    c. The patient completed independent COG wheel exercises without pain.

    d. The patient was able to complete all reps and sets of her exercises today.

13. Identify the statement that would **NOT** be appropriate for the subjective section of the SOAP note.

   a. The patient's father stated that she did not sleep well last night.

   b. The patient stated that her pain prior to exercising was a 5/10 on the VRS.

   c. The patient was able to increase the weights for hip flexion from 3-lb to 5-lb.

   d. The patient stated that she was able to walk to her mailbox today.

14. Place an "S," "O," "A," or "P" next to each statement to represent the section of the SOAP note in which the statement would be placed.

   1. _____ The patient's daughter said that she is going to buy him a shower chair when he is discharged from the hospital.

   2. _____ The patient's daughter said she is going to buy him some new towels when he is discharged from the rehab center.

   3. _____ The patient was able to stand independently next to the sink to brush his teeth (~10 minutes)

   4. _____ The patient became agitated during the treatment session and refused to finish his exercises.

   5. _____ Patient's Ⓡ UE shld. flex. = 120°.

   6. _____ Patient increased Ⓡ UE shld. flex. since last treatment session by ~10°.

   7. _____ Patient now able to reach items on highest kitchen shelf.

   8. _____ Patient will walk independently 3 yards by Thursday.

   9. _____ Patient will be seen by nutritionist on Monday.

   10. _____ Patient will have her son bring her to therapy on Friday.

15. Some of the following statements are incorrect. Identify the correct statements by rewriting them and rewrite the incorrect statements to reflect the correction.

   Dx: 6-year-old male with Type 2 Spinal Muscular Atrophy.

   S: Pt.'s parents state that they would like their son to have the best life possible. Pt.'s parents also state that they want him to be included in all the same activities as the other children his age.

   O: ROM: all within normal limits. Strength: pt. has a 1–2 in some muscle groups, right is stronger that the left UE. Tone: flaccid. Alignment: not tested. Quality of movement: is dependent in all movement while in the bed or in a seated position. Pt. is unable to roll or sit without max assist. Pt. is unable to use the joystick on his power wheelchair. Automatic reactions: not tested. Functional skills: not tested. Adaptive equipment: pw w/c, padded wooden adjustment chair, TV pillow, jogging stroller, lap desk for eating, laptop computer, bath chair, custom made table for w/c, wooden ramp, seatbelt, light plastic cup.

A: Pt. will benefit from physical therapy to improve his quality of life.

P: Cont. physical therapy 3X/wk for 6 wk for ROM training and hand-eye coordination training.

—Signed, One Confused PTA

_____

_____

_____

_____

_____

_____

_____

_____

_____

_____

_____

_____

_____

_____

_____

_____

_____

_____

_____

_____

_____

_____

_____

_____

16. Write a SOAP note based on the following information:

Use today's date. This is a daily progress note.

Pt. Name:	<u>John Simon, age 81</u>
Dx:	ESRD, vision loss, left BKA, CHF, and depression.

Your supervising PT told you that she did a supervisory visit with Mr. Simon this morning, and she wants you, the PTA, to continue to see this pt. twice a day in his hospital room to maintain his ROM and increase his UE strength. The PT wants you to end each session by getting him into his w/c so the nurse's aide can walk him down the hall and into a small courtyard outside.

You walk into Mr. Simon's room and find him asleep, so you gently shake his shoulder to wake him up. You tell him that you are there for his PT, and he says he will try to do it but he is very tired today.

You begin the treatment session by asking Mr. Simon if you can raise the head of his bed so that he will be in a sitting position, and he says OK. After you have him sitting up, you ask him to raise both of his arms up above his head. He raises his arms, but his elbows are still bent at a 90° angle. You have him repeat this 5 times. Then you ask him if he can hold both arms straight out in front of him while you count to 5. He does it 3 times, but the last 2 times he could only hold it for 3 seconds. You then have him hold his arms in front of him again and ask him to do bicep curls on each side, for 10 times. He still lacks about 20° of full elbow ext. You ask him to straighten out his elbows, but he can't do so. You do PROM to get him to full ext. and hold it for 45 seconds, repeating it 5 times.

You perform a foot check of his LE and see that everything looks good and healthy. You hold onto his foot and ask him to bring it up toward his bottom. He does it 10 times. You then ask Mr. Simon if he can sit up at the edge of the bed (you have been working with him on this skill). He again states that he is very tired but that he will try. He moves his bottom over to the edge of the bed and puts his leg over the edge. He then sits there for about 30 seconds to catch his breath. You already have the w/c next to the bed with the brakes on, so you tell him where it is and that you will help him get into it. He stands on his leg and puts about 50% of his weight on your shoulders. You then do a pivot transfer and lower him into the chair. At this time, the nurse's aide walks into the room to take Mr. Simon to the courtyard.

As the three of you are walking out of the room, you tell Mr. Simon that he did well and that you will be back in the afternoon to see him again. The nurse's aide states that Mr. Simon will be having his dialysis early today because a specialist is coming to see him at 4:00 p.m. You make a note in the chart regarding this visit and realize that you will not be able to see Mr. Simon again today because you are scheduled to attend an inservice training being led by a student PTA right after lunch.

_____

_____

_____

_____

_____

_____

_____

17. Write a separate SOAP note based on the following **first** and **second** treatment sessions and the following the evaluation information:

Evaluation Notes:

Name: Bill Smith   **Age:**   48 yrs. old

Past Med. Hx: Three years ago, he had 3 seizures and had been dx'd with a brain tumor. Pt. reported that he had chemotherapy and radiation and had been monitored for 2 years. A year ago, the tumor grew back and he had surgery to remove it. Pt. had a second surgery 2 months ago to remove necrotic tissue following radiation.

Pt. told PT and PTA the following information during the initial evaluation:

1. That he had physical therapy after the first surgery and had been able to jog.

2. He had inpatient physical therapy after the 2nd surgery for 2 weeks but did not continue it in an outpatient setting.

3. Complains of left-sided weakness.

4. Reported that he has intermittent MRIs to monitor his brain for additional tumors.

5. Reported that his condition has limited his ADLs, such as working on his car, driving, hunting, fishing, doing laundry, and cleaning his house.

6. Reported that he can dress, bathe, brush his teeth, shave, and feed himself independently.

7. No complaints of pain.

8. Reported that he does fall frequently, about 2X/month.

9. Reported that he has 3 steps into his house, which he can do independently with a quad cane. However, someone must hold the screen door open for him.

10. Pt. lives with his 20-year-old daughter who helps with ADLs, when needed.

11. Patient reports that he has been receiving chemotherapy for the past year for 5 days/month. Pt. reported that this causes him to get very fatigued. He said that the doctor told him the chemotherapy will have to be continued for the next 1–2 years.

12. Pt. reports that he is on 2 different seizure meds. and takes oxycodone as needed for pain.

13. Pt. reported that his goals are to increase his function, to be able to drive and work on his care, to be able to perform activities such as doing the dishes, and increased independence in ADLs.

You observed the following during the evaluation:

1. Pt. walks with a quad cane in place on the right side.

2. Pt. has a slow gait pattern with decreased arm swing on the left side.

3. Demonstrates increased left hip flexion, knee flexion, and dorsiflexion during gait with left lower extremity externally rotated and decreased toe clearance on the left during swing phase.

4. ROM.

LEs: Demonstrated full passive range of motion in both sides of the hip and knee. Left ankle AROM dorsiflexion is 110° and PROM dorsiflexion is 120°.

UEs: Right upper extremity is normal, left upper extremity is as follows:

Shld. flex.= 65°   Shld. abd = 75°

Elbow flex. = 135°   Elbow ext. = -5°

Pt. demonstrated no active movement in the left wrist or hand.

5. Strength:

Hip flex.	R = 3+/5	L = 3/5
Hip abd	R = 4+/5	L = 3–/5
Knee ext.	R = WNL	L = 4/5
Knee flex.	R = WNL	L = 3-/5
Dorsiflexion	R = WNL	L = 1/5
Plantar flexion	R = WNL	L = 1/5
Ankle inversion	R = WNL	L = WNL
Eversion	R = WNL	L = 0/5
Shld. flex.	R = WNL	L = 2/5
Abduction	R = WNL	L = WNL
Shld. shrug	R = WNL	L = 3-/5
Elbow ext.	R = WNL	L = 5/5
Elbow flex.	R = WNL	L = 4-/5
Wrist flexion	R = WNL	L = 1/5
Wrist ext.	R = WNL	L = 1/5

Here are some goals your PT told you to include in the plan of care:

STGs: To be completed in 3 weeks:

1. Increase wrist and ankle strength.

2. Instruct pt. in HEP for increased strength and ROM.

3. Increase left ankle PROM.

LTGs: To be completed in 8–10 weeks:

1. Increase left UE and LE strength.

2. Increase left ankle dorsiflexion AROM to 0°.

3. Increase left shld. AROM in flex. and abd to 100°.

4. Pt. will report he has not fallen in 1 month.

5. Pt. will be able to ascend 3 steps into his house and open the screen door independently.

6. Pt. will be able to do dishes using both hands.

7. Pt. will report that he is able to drive short distances in an automatic car.

8. Pt. will walk 50 ft independently without an assistive device.

The PT informs you that the pt. will be seen 1–2X/week for 2.5 months.

Notes from 1st treatment session:

Pt. stated that he has been doing the HEP he had been given after his initial evaluation. He stated that he can move his left ankle independently more now and has less stiffness in his left hand. During the first treatment session, you perform the following:

1. AROM ex. with left wrist and ankle, pt. demonstrated some independent ext. rotation in left wrist and increased PROM of dorsiflexion to –15°.

2. You also performed some resistance training in the left UE with a 1-lb. weight. Pt. was able to perform 5 shld. shrugs and w each of shld. flex and abd.

3. You did short arc quads on the left side with a 2-lb ankle weight; the pt. was able to complete 8 repetitions.

4. You finished with massage to the left UE.

5. You decide that you will talk to the PT about ordering a spasticity splint for his left hand.

Write a SOAP note based on the first treatment session.

_____

_____

_____

_____

_____

_____

_____

_____

_____

_____

_____

Notes from 2nd treatment session:

1. Told the pt. that the PT has ordered him a special splint for his hand and that it should arrive before his next tx session.

2. AROM ex. to left UE and LE. Pt. demonstrated increased AROM in dorsiflexion and was able to flex his wrist about 15°.

3. Resistance training to UEs and LEs using same amount of weight as first tx. session, but this time he did 10 shld. shrugs, 5 each of shld. flex. and ext. and 10 SAQ.

4. Pt. was able to ambulate about 5 steps without his quad cane twice today.

5. Session was completed with massage to left UE.

Write a SOAP note based on the second treatment session.

_____

_____

_____

_____

_____

_____

_____

_____

_____

_____

_____

_____

_____

_____

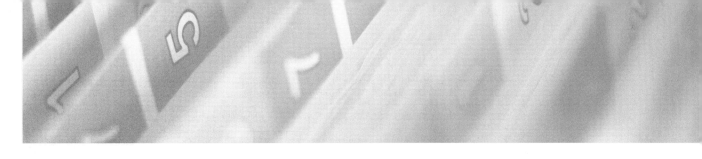

BIBLIOGRAPHY

1. American Physical Therapy Association. (2003). *Guide to physical therapist practice*. Alexandria, VA: APTA.
2. American Physical Therapy Association and the Section on Pediatrics. (1990). Individualized educational program and individualized family service plan. In K. D. Martin (Ed.), *Physical therapy practice in educational environments: Policies and guidelines* (p. 6.1). Alexandria, VA: APTA.
3. American Physical Therapy Association Terminology Task Force of the Acute Care Section. (1999, January). Alexandria, VA: APTA.
4. Anderson, K., & Anderson, L. (1990). *Mosby's pocket dictionary of medicine, nursing, & allied health*. St. Louis: Mosby.
5. Baeten, A. M., et al. (1999). *Documenting physical therapy: The reviewer perspective*. Woburn, MA: Butterworth-Heinemann.
6. Bernstein, F., et al. (1987). Insurance reimbursement and the physical therapist: Documentation for outpatient physical therapy; Guidelines based on California state law. *Clinical Management in Physical Therapy, 2*, 28–33.
7. Brown, S. R. (1987). Physical therapy documentation—Part III. *The Pyramid, 17*, 2.
8. Cutone, J. (1994). One PTA's experience: Team collaboration in the school setting. *PT Magazine, 3*, 48.
9. Davis, C., & Lippert, L. (September 1994). Facilitators: Reaching agreement about key content areas in PTA curricula. PTA educators colloquium, Minneapolis. Proceedings to be published by American Physical Therapy Association, Alexandria, VA.
10. Delitto, A., & Snyder-Mackler, L. (1995). The diagnostic process. Examples in orthopedic physical therapy. *Physical Therapy, 3*, 203.
11. Duncan, P. (April, 1995). *Balance dysfunction and motor control theory*. Workshop notes, College of St. Scholastica, Duluth, MN.
12. Erickson, M., & McKnight, B. (2005). *Documentation basics: A guide for the physical therapist assistant*. Thorofare, NJ: Slack..
13. Esposto, L. (1993). Applying functional outcome assessment to Medicare documentation. In D. L. Stewart and S. H. Abeln (Eds.), *Documenting functional outcomes in physical therapy*. St. Louis: Mosby.
14. Feitelberg, S. B. (Presenter). (1991, March). *A systematic approach to documentation: The basis for successful reimbursement*. American Rehabilitation Educational Network (AREN) teleconference.
15. Government Affairs Department. (1992). *Physical therapy practice without referral: "direct access."* Alexandria, VA: American Physical Therapy Association.
16. Guccione, A. (2007). Functional assessment. In S. B. O'Sullivan and J. J.Schmitz (Eds.), *Physical rehabilitation, assessment, and treatment*. Philadelphia: FA Davis.
17. Hebert, L. (1981). Basics of Medicare documentation for physical therapy. *Clinical Management, 1*(3), 13.
18. Hill, J. R. (1987). *The problem-oriented approach to physical therapy care*. Alexandria, VA: American Physical Therapy Association.
19. Jette, A. M. (1993). Using health-related quality of life measures in physical therapy outcomes research. *Physical Therapy, 8*, 528.
20. Langley, G. B., & Sheppeard, H. (1985). The visual analogue scale: Its use in pain measurement. *RheumatologyInternational, 5*, 145.
21. Lunning, S. (Presenter). (1994, May). *Opportunity or chaos? Prepare for the future in physical therapy*. Minnesota Chapter American Physical Therapy Association Peer Review Workshop, Virginia, MN.
22. Lupi-Williams, F. A. (1983). The PTA role and function: An analysis in three parts. Part 1: education. *Clinical Management Physical Therapy, 3*, 3.
23. McGuire, D. B. (1984). The measurement of clinical pain. *Nursing Research, 3*, 152.
24. Melzack, R. (1975). The McGill pain questionnaire: Major properties and scoring methods. *Pain, 1*, 277.
25. Moffat, M. (1995, Fall). Foreword. *Journal of Physical Therapy Education, 9*, 35.
26. Montgomery, P., & Connolly, B. (1991). *Motor control and physical therapy: Theoretical framework, practical application* (1st ed.). Hixson, TN: Chattanooga Group.
27. Nagi, S. Z. (1969). *Disability and rehabilitation*. Columbus, OH: Ohio University Press.
28. Ransford, A., et al. (1976). The pain drawing as an aid to the psychologic evaluation of patients with low-back pain. *Spine, 1*, 127.
29. Rogers, J. (1991, July/August). PTA utilization: The big picture. *Clinical Management in Physical Therapy, 11*(4), 8.
30. Rose, S. (1989). Diagnosis: Defining the term. *Physical Therapy, 69*, 162.
31. Stewart, D.L., & Abeln, S. H. (1993). *Documenting functional outcomes in physical therapy*. St. Louis: Mosby.
32. Swanson, G. (1995, December). *Essentials for the future of physical therapy, every therapist's concern*. A Continuing Education 30. Course. Minnesota Chapter American Physical Therapy Association, Duluth, MN.
33. Task Force on Standards for Measurement in Physical Therapy. (1991). Standards for tests and measurements in physical therapy practice. *Physical Therapy, 71*, 589.
34. Terminology Task Force of the Acute Care Section of American Physical Therapy Association. (1999, January). *Common terminology*. Decatur, GA.

35. Thomas, C. L. (Ed.). (2005). *Taber's cyclopedic medical dictionary* (17th ed.). Philadelphia: FA Davis.

36. World Health Organization. (2001). *International classification of functioning, disability, and health.* Geneva, Switzerland.

37. World Health Organization. (1980). *International classification of impairments, disabilities, and handicaps.* Geneva, Switzerland.

38. Yaeger, J. (1990). *Effective listening techniques.* Notes from Mgt 503, Oral Communication. Masters in Management Program. College of St. Scholastica, Duluth, MN.

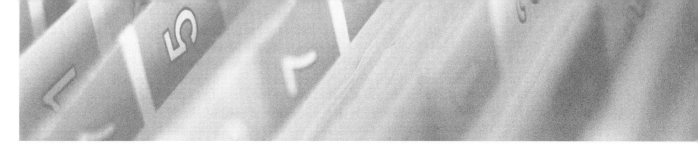

GLOSSARY

A

Accountable: Responsible, capable of explaining oneself.

Accredit: To supply with credentials or authority.

Accreditation: Granting of approval to an institution by an official review board after the institution has met specific requirements.

Adhesive capsulitis: A condition characterized by adhesions and shortening or tightening of the connective tissue sleeve that encases a joint.

Ambulate: To walk about.

American Physical Therapy Association: Professional organization representing the physical therapy profession, the occupation consisting of professionals and technicians trained to provide the medical rehabilitative service of physical therapy.

Antalgic: Painful or indicating the presence of pain.

Anterior joint capsule: Front portion of the joint connective tissue sleeve.

Assessment: Measurement, quantification, or placement of a value or label on something; assessment is often confused with evaluation; an assessment results from the act of assessing.*

Ataxia: Condition characterized by impaired ability to coordinate movement. Ataxic gait is a staggering, uncoordinated walk.

Athetosis: Condition characterized by impaired movement, often marked by slow, writhing movements of the hands.†

Audit: Examination of records to check accuracy and compliance with professional standards.

Authenticate: To verify, to prove, to establish as worthy of belief.

Autonomy: Independent functioning, ability to self-govern.

B

Balance: Ability to maintain the body in equilibrium with gravity in either a static or dynamic process.†

Biomechanics: Study of mechanical forces and their interaction with living organisms, especially the human body.

C

Circumduct: To move the joint in a circular manner.

Clinical decision: Determination that relates to direct patient care, indirect patient care, acceptance of patients for treatment, and whether patients should be referred to other practitioners.‡ A diagnosis that leads a therapist to take an action is a form of a clinical decision; clinical decisions result in actions; when direct supporting evidence for clinical decisions is lacking, such decisions are based on clinical opinions.

Cognition: Act or process of knowing, including both awareness and judgment.†

Collaborate: To work together, to cooperate.

Concentric contraction: Muscle contraction that moves the muscle from a resting, lengthened position to a shortened position; a muscle contraction in which the insertion and origin move closer together.

Continuum: A continuous extent, succession, or whole.

Coordination: Muscle action of the appropriate intensity, timing, and sequencing to produce a smooth, controlled, purposeful movement.

Compensation: The ability of an individual with a disability to perform a task, either by using the impaired limb with an adapted approach or by using the unaffected limb to perform the task; an approach to rehabilitation in which the patient is taught to adapt to and offset a residual disability.[†]

Contracture: A condition of fixed, high resistance to passive stretching that results from fibrosis and shortening of tissues that support muscles or joints[†].

Criteria: Requirements, standards, rules.

Cyanosis: A bluish or purplish discoloration of the skin due to a severe oxygen deficiency.[†]

D

Data: Raw information, uninterpreted information organized for analysis or used as the basis for a decision.

Débridement: Excision of contused or necrotic tissue from the surface of a wound.[†]

Diagnosis: A label encompassing a cluster of signs and symptoms, syndromes, or categories. It is the decision reached as a result of the diagnostic process, which includes (1) evaluating the data obtained during the examination, (2) organizing it into cluster syndromes or categories, and (3) interpreting it.[†]

Direct access: Legislation that enables the consumer to enter the medical care system by going directly to a physical therapist. The patient needing physical therapy treatment does not need to be referred to a physical therapist by a physician.

Disability: The inability to engage in age-specific, gender-related, and sex-specific roles in a particular social context and physical environment.[§]

Discharge evaluation: A document written by the PT containing recommendations and decisions about future treatment when treatment is terminated by the PT.

Discharge summary: A document that may be written by the PTA stating the treatments provided and the status of the patient at the time of discharge. If this document contains recommendations or decisions about future treatment, it is considered an evaluation and must be written by the PT.

Documentation: Written information supplying proof, a written record, supporting references.

Dysarthria: A motor disorder that results in impairment of motor speech mechanisms.[†]

Dysphagia: Difficulty in swallowing.[†]

Dyspnea: Shortness of breath; subjective difficulty or distress in breathing frequently manifested by rapid, shallow breaths; usually associated with serious diseases of the heart or lungs.[†]

Duration: Period of time in which something persists or exists.

E

Eccentric contraction: A muscle contraction that moves the muscle from a shortened position to its lengthened or resting position; muscle contraction in which the insertion and origin move away from each other.

Edema: Swelling; accumulation of fluid in the tissues.

Efficacy: Effectiveness, ability to achieve results.

Episode of care: All physical therapy services that are (1) provided by a physical therapist or under the direction and supervision of a physical therapist, (2) provided in an unbroken sequence, and (3) related to the physical therapy interventions for a given condition or problem or related to a request from the patient/client, family, or other health-care provider.[§]

Erythema: Describing an abnormal redness of the skin.[†]

Evaluation: Judgment based on a measurement; often confused with assessment and examination; evaluations are judgments of the value or worth of something. A dynamic process in which the physical therapist makes clinical judgments based on data gathered during the examination.[§]

Examination: Test or a group of tests used for the purpose of obtaining measurements or data.[*] The process of obtaining a history, performing relevant systems reviews, and selecting and administering specific tests and measurements.[§]

Extension: Movement of a joint in which the angle between the two adjoining bones increases.

Exudation: Process of expressing material through a wound, usually characterized as oozing.

F

Facilitate: To enhance or help an action or function.

Femur: Thigh bone.

Flexion: Movement of a joint in which the angle decreases between the two adjoining bones.

Fractured: Broken. Typically refers to broken bones.

Fremitus: Sensation felt when placing a hand on a body part that vibrates during speech or deep breathing.[†]

Frequency: Number of times something occurs, number of repetitions, number of treatment sessions.

Function: Those activities identified by an individual as essential to support physical, social, and psychological well-being and to create a personal sense of meaningful living.[†]

Functional limitation: Restriction of the ability to perform a physical action, activity, or task in an efficient, typically expected, or competent manner.[§]

G

Gait: Walking pattern; the manner in which a person walks.

Gait Patterns:[†]

Two-point gait: Assistive device and contralateral lower extremity advance and meet the floor simultaneously.

Three-point gait: Assistive devices and one weight-bearing lower extremity maintain contact with the floor.

Four-point gait: In sequential order of contact: the left crutch is advanced, followed by the right lower extremity, then the right crutch is advanced prior to the left lower extremity.

Swing-to gait: Pattern in which both crutches (or other assistive device) are advanced, and then bilateral lower extremities advance parallel to the plane of the assistive device.

Swing-through gait: Pattern in which both crutches (or other assistive device) are advanced, and then bilateral lower extremities advance anterior to the placement of the device.

Tandem walk: Heel-to-toe pattern in which the heel is placed in front of the toe of the opposite extremity; pattern is repeated with each lower extremity.

Braiding/grapevine-gait: Pattern in which the left lower extremity is adducted anterior to the right lower extremity, the right lower extremity is abducted, the left lower extremity is adducted posterior to the right lower extremity, and the right lower extremity is abducted to complete the sequence. Sequence may be repeated with the right lower extremity initiating.

Girth: Distance around something, circumference.

Goal: Those statement(s) that define the patient's expected level of performance at the end of the rehabilitation process; the functional outcomes of therapy, indicating the amount of independence, supervision, or assistance required and the equipment or environmental adaptation necessary to ensure adequate performance. Desired outcomes may be stated as long-term or short-term as determined by the needs of the patient and the setting.[†]

Goniometry: Procedure for measuring the range-of-motion angles of a joint.

H

Hamstrings: Common name for the group of three muscles located on the posterior thigh.

Handicap: As defined by the World Health Organization, the disadvantage resulting from an impairment or disability that limits or prevents fulfillment of a role that is normal, depending on age, sex, and social/cultural factors. Handicap describes the social and economic roles of impaired or disabled persons that place them at a disadvantage when compared with others (e.g., inability to use public transportation, inability to work, social isolation).[†]

Health status: Level of an individual's physical, mental, affective, and social functions. Health status is an element of well-being.[†]

Hemianopsia: Loss of vision in one-half of the visual field of one or both eyes.[†]

Hip extensors: Common name for the group of muscles that produce extension motion of the hip joint.

Homonymous hemianopsia: Defective vision or blindness affecting the right or left half of the visual fields of both eyes.[†]

Hypertonus: Excessive muscle tone or prolonged muscle contraction.

I

Impairment: A loss or abnormality of physiological, psychological, or anatomical structure or function.[§]

Incident: Distinct occurrence; an event inconsistent with usual routine or treatment procedure; an accident.

Incident report: Documentation required when an unusual event occurs in a clinical or medical facility.

Individual educational program: Written statement outlining the goals and objectives for the services provided to meet a physically disabled child's educational needs.

Informed consent: Permission or agreement for medical treatment on the basis of knowledge of all the information about the treatment.

Initial and mid swing: Portions of the walking pattern when the heel and then the toes leave the ground and the leg swings to the point where the hip is at 0° flexion or extension.

Instrumental activities of daily living (IADL): Activities that are important components of maintaining independent living (e.g., shopping, cooking).[†]

Internship: Period of time during which a medical professional in training provides clinical care under supervision.

Intervention: The purposeful and skilled interaction of the physical therapist with the patient/client and, when appropriate, with other individuals involved in care, using various methods and techniques to produce changes in the patient's/client's condition.[§]

J

Joint Commission on Accreditation of Healthcare Organizations: Agency with the responsibility to ensure that hospitals and medical centers follow federal and state regulations and meet the standards necessary for the provision of safe and appropriate health care.

Joint integrity: Conformance of the joints to expected anatomical, biomechanical, and kinematic norms.[†]

Joint mobility: Ability to move a joint; takes into account the structure and shape of the joint surface as well as characteristics of tissue surrounding the joint.[†]

K

Kinesthesia: The awareness of the body's or a body part's movement.[†]

L

Laceration: Torn, jagged wound.

Lag: To fall behind, not keep up, develop slowly, weaken, or slacken.

Lower extremity: Area that includes the thigh, lower leg, and foot.

M

Medicaid: Federally funded, state-administered health insurance for eligible individuals with low income who are too young to qualify for Medicare.

Medical diagnosis: Identification of a systemic disease or disorder on the basis of the findings from a physician's examination and diagnostic tests.

Medicare: Federally funded national health insurance for qualifying persons older than 65.

Mobilization techniques: Manual techniques or procedures used by physical therapy professionals to increase the range of motion of a joint.

Modality: Method of therapy or treatment procedure.

Motor function: The ability to learn or demonstrate the skilful and efficient assumption, maintenance, modification, and control of voluntary postures and movement patterns.[†]

Fine: Refers to relatively delicate movements, such as using a fork or tying a shoelace.

Gross: Refers to larger-scale movements, such as assuming an upright position or carrying a bag.

Muscle spasms: Persistent, involuntary contractions of a muscle or certain groups of muscle fibers within the muscle.

Muscle tone:[†] The velocity-dependent resistance to stretch that muscle exhibits.

Flaccidity: Total loss of muscle tension or responsiveness to stimulation.

Hypotonia: Reduced muscular tension with a slowed response to stimulation.

Hypertonia: Increased muscular tension resulting in resistance to movement, with increased speed and effort of movement.

Mild: A slight resistance to movement, with full ROM when movement is performed slowly (not apparent at rest).

Moderate: A resistance to movement with limitation to the variety and smoothness or response to stimulation that is affected by positioning and the speed of movement.

Severe: Observed posturing at rest, with limitation in ROM and resistance to movement regardless of the position or speed of stimulation.

N

Nagi Model: This model provides a definitive summary of an active pathology with the relationship to the resulting impairment, functional limitation, and disability.

Negligence: State of being extremely careless or lacking in concern.

Neuromusculoskeletal: Pertaining to the nervous system, the muscular system, and the skeletal system.

O

Objective: Measurable behavioral statement of an expected response or outcome; something worked toward or striven for; a statement of direction or desired achievement that guides actions and activities.[†]

Occupational therapist: Trained health-care professional who provides occupational therapy.

Occupational therapy assistant: Trained health-care technician who provides occupational therapy under the supervision of an occupational therapist.

Orthopedics: Branch of medicine devoted to the study and treatment of the skeletal system and its joints, muscles, and associated structures.

Orthostatic hypotension: Lowering of systolic blood pressure >10 mm Hg with a change of body position from supine to erect, which may or may not be accompanied by clinical signs.[†]

Outcomes: Outcomes are the result of patient/client management. They are related to remediation of functional limitations and disabilities, primary or secondary prevention, and optimization of patient/client satisfaction.[†]

Outcomes analysis: A systematic examination of patient/client outcomes in relation to selected patient/client variables; outcomes analysis may be used in a quality assessment, economic analysis or practice, and other processes.[†]

Oxygen saturation: The degree to which oxygen is present in a particular cell, tissue, organ, or system.[†]

P

Palpable: Able to be felt or touched; as in touching with the hands.

Parameters: Limits or boundaries; a value or constant used to describe or measure a set of data representing a physiological function or system.

Paraparesis: Partial paralysis or extreme weakness.

Pathokinesiologic: Pertaining to the study of movements related to a given disorder.

Pathological: Pertaining to a condition that is caused by or involves a disease.

Pathology: Study of the characteristics, causes, and effects of disease.

Percussion (diagnostic): Procedure in which the clinician taps a body part manually or with an instrument to estimate its density.[†]

Perseveration: Involuntary and pathological persistence of the same verbal response or motor activity regardless of the type of stimulus or its duration.[†]

Physical function: Fundamental component of health status describing the state of those sensory and motor skills necessary for mobility, work, and recreation.[†]

Physical therapist assistant: A technically educated health-care provider who assists the physical therapist in the provision of physical therapy. The physical therapist assistant, under the direction and supervision of the physical therapist, is the only paraprofessional who provides physical therapy interventions. The physical therapist assistant is a graduate of a physical therapist assistant degree program accredited by the Commission on Accreditation in Physical Therapy Education (CAPTE).[§]

Physical therapy: The treatment of impairments and functional limitations by physical means, such as exercise, education and training, heat, light, electricity, water, cold, ultrasound, massage, and manual therapy to improve or restore the patient's ability to function in his or her environment. Physical therapy is provided by trained persons who have graduated from accredited physical therapy and physical therapist assistant programs.

Physical Therapy Practice Act: Legislation in each state that defines and regulates the practice or provision of physical therapy services.

Physical therapy problem: Identification of the neuromusculoskeletal dysfunction and resulting functional limitation that is treatable with physical therapy.

Physician assistants: Trained technicians providing medical care under the supervision of a physician.

Plan of care: Statements that specify the anticipated long-term and short-term goals and the desired outcomes, predicted level of optimal improvement, specific interventions to be used, duration and frequency of the intervention required to reach the goals and outcomes, and criteria for discharge.[†]

Prevention:[†]
Primary: Preventing disease in a susceptible or potentially susceptible population through specific measures, such as general health-promotion efforts.
Secondary: Decreasing duration of illness, severity of disease, and sequelae through early diagnosis and prompt intervention.
Tertiary: Limiting the degree of disability and promoting rehabilitation and restoration of function in patients with chronic and irreversible diseases.

Problem-oriented: Based on or directed toward the problem, as when the medical record is organized around the identification of the medical problems.

Prognosis: Determination of the level of optimal improvement that might be attained by the patient/client and the amount of time needed to reach that level.[†]

Proprioception: The reception of stimuli from within the body; includes position sense and kinesthesia.[†]

Prone: Horizontal with the face downward. Opposite of supine.

Psoriasis: Common, chronic, inheritable skin disorder characterized by circumscribed red patches covered by thick, dry, silvery, adherent scales.

Q

Quadriparesis (tetraplegia): Partial paralysis or extreme weakness of arms, legs, and trunk resulting from injury to spinal nerves in the cervical spine.

Quality assurance: Title of the department, usually in health-care facilities, that reviews medical charts to identify when regulations and standards are not being met or when unsafe or inappropriate medical care is being provided.

Quality assurance committee: Group that performs chart reviews.

R

Range of motion:[†] The space, distance, or angle through which movement occurs at a joint or a series of joints.
Passive (PROM): 100% therapist/assistant-performed movement through the available excursion of the joint or body segment.
Active (AROM): 100% self-performed movement through the available excursion of the joint or body segment.
Active assistive (AAROM): Partial self-performed movement with external assistance provided to complete the desired available excursion of the joint or body segment.

Rehabilitation facilities: Clinics or institutions that provide rehabilitation services, such as physical therapy, occupational therapy, speech pathology, psychological services, social services, orthotics and prosthetics, and patient and family education.

Rehabilitation types:[†]

Acute: Term used by some sources to denote intense rehabilitation in an inpatient rehabilitation facility or designated unit.

Comprehensive: Rehabilitation involving a full array of rehabilitation services and disciplines.

Intense: Generally interpreted to mean rehabilitation involving 3 or more hours of acute physical, occupational, psychological, or speech and language therapy per day, 5 or more days per week.

Rehabilitation hospital: Free-standing hospital that is organized and staffed to provide intense and comprehensive inpatient rehabilitation.

Rehabilitation unit: Distinct part of an acute care hospital or skilled nursing facility that is organized and staffed to provide intense and comprehensive inpatient rehabilitation.

Subacute care: Goal-oriented, comprehensive inpatient care designed for an individual who has had an acute illness, injury, or exacerbation of a disease process and is rendered immediately after, or instead of, acute hospitalization.

Reimbursement: Payment for services.

Release-of-information form: Document that the patient signs to give permission for the person(s) named in the document to receive information about the patient's medical condition and treatment.

Reliable: Dependable, reproducible.

Retrospective: Looking back on, contemplating, or directed to the past.

Rule of confidentiality: A principle that information about patients should not be revealed to anyone not authorized to receive the information.

S

Signs: Characteristics or indications of disease or dysfunction determined by objective tests, measurements, or observations.

Source-oriented: Organized around the source of the information, as when the medical record is organized according to the various disciplines providing and documenting the care.

Speech pathologist: Trained professional who diagnoses and treats abnormalities in speech.

Status quo: No change in a specified state or condition.

Strengthening:[†]

Active: Form of strength-building exercise in which the therapist applies resistance through the range of motion of active movement.

Assistive: Form of strength-building exercise in which the therapist assists the patient/client through the available range of motion.

Resistive: Any form of active exercise in which a dynamic or static muscular contraction is resisted by an outside force. The external force can be applied manually or mechanically.

Isometric exercise: Active contraction of a muscle or group of muscles against a stable force without joint movement.

Isokinetic exercise: Active movement performed at an established fixed speed against an accommodating resistance.

Symptoms: Subjective characteristics or indications of disease or dysfunction as perceived by the patient.

Systemic: Pertaining to the whole body.

Systems review: A brief or limited examination that provides additional information about the patient's general health to help the physical therapist formulate a diagnosis and select an intervention program.[†]

T

Tactile: Pertaining to the sense of touch.

Third-party payer: Medical reimbursement agency, such as Medicare, Medicaid, managed care organizations, indemnity insurers, and businesses that contract for services. Each type of payer has its own reimbursement policies.

Transfers/Position:[†]

Dependent transfer: Patient/client relies totally on external support for transfer; exerts no physical assistance in transfer.

Sliding board/transfer board: Patient/client transfers with assistance of board placed under ischial tuberositates; board bridges two opposing surfaces.

Depression transfer: Patient/client transfers by depressing scapulae with upper extremity pressure against surface and lifting pelvis laterally or anteroposteriorly.

Stand pivot: Patient/client transfers by pushing to stand and pivoting with one or both lower extremities.

Supported sitting: Sitting position maintained with external support and/or use of the patient's/client's upper extremities.

Unsupported sitting: Sitting position maintained without external support or use of the patient's/client's upper extremities.

Quadruped: Position where weight-bearing occurs on extended upper extremities and on flexed hips/knees; upper extremities placed at 90° should flexion with 0–10° abduction and full elbow extension, and lower extremities are placed on 90° hip-knee flexion with lower legs resting parallel to floor.

Long sitting: Sitting with hips at 90° angle and bilateral lower extremities extended fully on a supported surface.

U

Ulcers:[†]

Stage I: Nonblanchable erythema of intact skin reversible with intervention.

Stage II: Tissue loss involving the epidermis and dermis that may present as an abrasion, blister, or a shallow crater, with a wound base moist and pink, painful, free of necrotic tissue.

Stage III: Damage or actual necrosis of subcutaneous tissue that may extend down to but not through the fascial layer; may include necrotic tissue; wound base not usually painful.

Stage IV: Tissue loss extending to the level of bone, muscle, tendon, or to a supporting structure; involves necrotic tissue; wound base usually not painful.

V

Vital signs: Measurements of pulse rate, respiration rate, body temperature, and blood pressure.

W

Weight-bearing status:[†]

Non-weight bearing (NWB): No weight on involved extremity.

Toe-touch/touchdown/foot-flat weight-bearing (TTWB, TDWB, FFW): Extremity may rest on floor (is unloaded); negligible weight is placed on extremity. Status used primarily for balance or stability during gait and transfers.

Partial weight-bearing (PWB): Prescribed, measured percentage of weight is allowed.

Weight-bearing as tolerated (WBAT): As much weight as is tolerated within pain limits is allowed.

Full weight-bearing (FWB): 100% of body weight, with or without assistive devices, is allowed.

Workers' compensation: State- and business-funded health insurance that manages and funds medical care for persons injured on the job.

---

[*]Task Force on Standards for Measurement in Physical Therapy. (1991). Standards for tests and measurement in physical therapy practice. *Physical Therapy, 71,* 589.

[†]Task Force of the Acute Care Section on Terminology. APTA, Alexandria, VA. January 1999.

[‡]This definition is modified from that presented by Charles Magistro at a conference on Clinical Decision Making held under APTA auspices October 1988 in Lake of the Ozarks, MO.

[§]American Physical Therapy Association. (2003). *Guide to physical therapist practice* (2nd ed., Appendix 1). Alexandria, VA: APTA.

Appendix A

Abbreviations

A

ā	before
A	assessment
Ⓐ	assist
A/	active
AA/	active assist
AAA	abdominal aortic aneurysm
AAL	anterior axial line
AAROM	active assistive range of motion
abd/add	abduction/adduction
ABG	arterial blood gases
ABI	acquired brain injury
abn	abnormal
ac	before meals
ACA	anterior cerebral artery
AC joint	acromioclavicular joint
ACL	anterior cruciate ligament
ADA	American with Disabilities Act, American Diabetes Association
ADL	activities of daily living
ad lib	at discretion
AE	above elbow
afib	atrial fibrillation
AFO	ankle foot orthosis
AIDS	acquired immune deficiency syndrome
AIIS	anterior inferior iliac spine
A/K	above knee
AKA	above knee amputation
AKS	arthroscopic knee surgery
A-line	arterial line
ALS	amyotrophic lateral sclerosis
AKFO	ankle knee foot orthosis
am, a.m.	morning, before noon
AMA	against medical advice
amb.	ambulation
amt	amount
ANS	autonomic nervous system
ant	anterior
ante	before
A-P	anterior-posterior
appts	appointments
APTA	American Physical Therapy Association
ARC	AIDS-related complex
ARD	adult respiratory distress
ARDS	adult respiratory distress syndrome

ARF	acute renal failure
AROM	active range of motion
ASAP	as soon as possible
ASCVD	arteriosclerotic cardiovascular disease
ASD	arterial septal defect
ASHD	arteriosclerotic heart disease
ASIS	anterior superior iliac spine
assist.	assistance
ATNR	asymmetrical tonic neck reflex
A-V	arterio-venous
AVM	avascular necrosis
AVR	aortic valve replacement
AVS	arteriovenous shunt
ax. cr	axillary crutches

B

Ⓑ	bilateral, both
BBA	Balanced Budget Act of 1997
BBB	bundle branch block
BBFA	both bone forearm (fractures)
b/c	because
BC/BS	Blue Cross/Blue Shield
BE	below elbow
bid	twice a day
bil.	bilateral
biw	twice a week
BK	below knee
BKA	below knee amputation
BLE	both lower extremities
BM	bowel movement
BOS	base of support
BP	blood pressure
BPD	bronchopulmonary dysplasia
BPF	bronchopleural fistula
BPM	beats per minute
BR	bedrest
B/S, B.S.	beside, bedside
BS	breath sounds, bowel sounds
BUE	both upper extremities
BUN	blood urea nitrogen

C

c̄	with
CA	carcinoma, cancer
CABG	coronary artery bypass graft
CAD	coronary artery disease
CAPTE	Commission on Accreditation for Physical Therapy Education
CARF	Commission on Accreditation of Rehabilitation Facilities
CAT	computerized axial tomography
CBC	complete blood count
C/C, C/Cs	chief complaint, chief complaints
cc	cubic centimeter
CCU	coronary care unit
C & DB	cough and deep breathing
CF	cystic fibrosis

CGA	contact guard assist
CHD	congenital heart disease, congenital hip dislocation
CHF	congestive heart failure
CHI	closed head injury
CiTx	cervical intermittent traction
cm	centimeter(s)
CMS	Center for Medicare and Medicaid Services
CMV	cytomegalovirus
CN	cranial nerve
CNS	central nervous system
c/o	complains of, complaint(s) of
CO	cardiac output
cont	continue
coord	coordination
COPD	chronic obstructive pulmonary disease
COTA	certified occupational therapist assistant
CP	compression pump, cerebral palsy
CPAP	continuous positive airway pressure
CPM	continuous passive motion machine
CPR	cardiopulmonary resuscitation
CPT	current procedural terminology, chest physical therapy
CRF	chronic renal failure
C-Section	cesarean section
CSF	cerebral spinal fluid
CT scan	computerized axial tomography
CVA	cerebral vascular accident
c/w	consistent with
CW	continuous wave
CX	cancel
CXR	chest x-ray

D

D_1, D_2	diagonal 1, diagonal 2 (proprioceptive neuromuscular facilitation [PNF] patterns)
d/c	discharged, discontinued
DEP	data, evaluation, performance goals
dept	department
DF	dorsiflexion
DI	diabetes insipidus
DIP	distal interphalangeal joint
DJD	degenerative joint disease
DM	diabetes mellitus
DME	durable medical equipment
DNR	do not resuscitate
DOA	dead on arrival
DOB	date of birth
DOD	date of discharge
DOE	dyspnea on exertion
DPT	diphtheria-pertussis-tetanus (vaccine)
DRGs	diagnosis related groups
drsg	dressing
DSD	dry sterile dressing
DTR	deep tendon reflex
DVT	deep venous thrombosis
Dx	diagnosis

E

ECF	extended care facility
ECG, EKG	electrocardiogram
EEG	electroencephalogram
elec.	electrical
EMG	electromyogram
ENT	ear, nose, throat
EOB	edge of bed
equip.	equipment
ER	emergency room
ERISA	Employer Retirement Income Security Act
E.S., E-stim	electrical stimulation
ESRD	end-stage renal disease
ETT	endotracheal tube
Ev, ev	eversion
Eval	evaluation
ex.	exercise
ext., /	extension

F

F	female, fair muscle strength grade
Ⓕ	father
FAQ	full arc quads
FAROM	functional active range of motion
FDA	Food and Drug Administration
FES	functional electrical stimulation
FIM	functional independence measure
flex. ✓	flexion
FOR	functional outcome report
FRC	functional residual capacity
ft	foot, feet
FTP	failure to progress
FTSG	full-thickness skin graft
F/U	follow up
FUO	fever unknown origin
FVC	forced vital capacity
FWB	full weight-bearing
FWW, fw/w	front wheeled walker
Fx, fx	fracture(d)

G

G	good (muscle strength, balance)
GA	gestational age
gastrocs	gastrocnemius muscles
GBS	Guillain Barré Syndrome
GCS	Glasgow Coma Scale
GERD	gastroesophageal reflux disease
GI	gastrointestinal
gluts.	gluteals
gm	gram
GMT	gross muscle test
GSW	gunshot wound
G-tube	gastrostomy tube
gt.	gait
GXT	graded exercise test

H

Ⓗ	husband
HBP	high blood pressure
HCFA	Health Care Financing Administration
H & P	history and physical
HA, H/A	headache
Hb, Hgb, HGB	hemoglobin
HCT, hct	hematocrit
HEENT	head, ears, eyes, nose, throat
Hemi	hemiplegia
Hep.	heparin
HEP	home exercise program
HHA	hand held assist, home health aide
HI	head injury
HIV	human immunodeficiency virus
HMO	health maintenance organization
HNP	herniated nucleus pulposus
h/o	history of
HO	heterotopic ossification
HOB	head of bed
HP	hot pack
HR	heart rate
hr	hour
h.s.	at bedtime
HS	hamstring(s)
ht.	height
HTN	hypertension
HWR	hardware removal
HX, Hx, hx	history

I

Ⓘ, indep.	independent
IBS	irritable bowel syndrome
ICBG	iliac crest bone graft
ICD-9	International Classification of Diseases
ICH	intracranial hemorrhage
ICIDH	International Classification of Impairments, Disabilities, and Handicaps
ICF	International Classification of Functioning, Disability, and Health
ICP	intracranial pressure
ICU	intensive care unit
IDDM	insulin dependent diabetes mellitus
I/E ratio	inspiratory/expiratory ratio
IEP	individual education program
IFC	extended care unit
IFSP	individual family service plan
ILV	independent lung ventilation
IM	intramuscular
IMV	intermittent mandatory ventilation
in.	inch(es)
inf.	inferior
int.	internal
IP	inpatient, interphalangeal
IPA	Individual Practice Association
IRDS	infant respiratory distress syndrome

IS	incentive spirometer
IV	intravenous

J

JAMA	Journal of the American Medical Association
JCAHO	Joint Commission on Accreditation of Healthcare Organizations
J-tube	jejunostomy tube
JRA	juvenile rheumatoid arthritis
jt.	joint

K

K	potassium
Kcal	kilocalories
kg	kilogram

L

L	liter
Ⓛ, lt.	left
L5	5th lumbar vertebra
LAQ	long arc quadriceps
lat.	lateral
lb	pound
LBBB	left bundle branch block
LBP	low back pain
LE, LEs	lower extremity, lower extremities
lg	large
lic.	license
LL	long leg braces
LLC	long leg cast
LLE	left lower extremity
LLL	left lower lobe
LMN	lower motor neuron
LOA	leave of absence
LOB	loss of balance
LOC	loss of or level of consciousness
LP	lumbar puncture
LPN	licensed practical nurse
LTC	long-term care
LTG	long-term goals
LUE	left upper extremity

M

M	male
Ⓜ	mother
m.	muscle
MAP	mean arterial pressure
m., mm.	muscle
max.	maximum
MCA	middle cerebral artery, motorcycle accident
MCO	managed care organization
M.D.	medical doctor, doctor of medicine
MD	muscular dystrophy
MDS	minimum data set
mech	mechanical
MED	minimal erythemal dose
meds.	medications

mg	milligram(s)
MH	moist heat
MHz	megahertz
MI	myocardial infarction
min	minute(s)
min.	minimum, minimal
mm	millimeter(s)
mm Hg	millimeters of mercury
MMT	manual muscle test
mo	month(s)
mod.	moderate
MP, MCP	metacarpophalangeal
MRI	magnetic resonance imaging
MRSA	methicillin resistant staph aureus
MS	multiple sclerosis
mtr.	motor
MVA	motor vehicle accident

N

N, nL	normal (muscle strength)
N/A	not applicable, not able
NAD	no acute distress
N & V	nausea and vomiting
NBQC	narrow-based quad cane
NCV	nerve conduction velocity
NDT	neurodevelopmental treatment
NEC	necrotizing enterocolitis
neg.	negative
NG	nasogastric
NICU	newborn intensive care unit
NIDDM	noninsulin dependent diabetes mellitus
NKA	no known allergies
nn	nerve
noc.	night, at night
NPO	nothing by mouth
NTT	nasotracheal tube
NWB	non–weight-bearing

O

O:	objective data
O_2 sat	oxygen saturation
OA	osteoarthritis
OASIS	outcome and assessment information sets
OB	obstetrics
OBS	organic brain syndrome
occ	occasional
OCD	obsessive compulsive disorder
OD	overdose
OGT	oral gastric tube
OM	otitis media
OOB	out of bed
OOT	out of town
OP	outpatient
OR	operating room
ORIF	open reduction, internal fixation
ortho	orthopedics

OT	occupational therapist
OTR	registered occupational therapist
oz	ounce(s)

P

p̄	post, after
P	poor (muscle strength, balance)
P/	passive
P:	plan (treatment plan)
PA	posterior/anterior
para	paraplegia
p.c.	after meals
PC	pressure control
PCA	patient controlled analgesia
PCL	posterior cruciate ligament
PCP	primary care physician
PCO$_2$	partial pressure of carbon dioxide
PD	postural drainage
PDA	patent ductus arteriosus
PDR	physician desk reference
PE	pulmonary embolus
peds	pediatrics
PEEP	positive end expiratory pressure
PF	plantar flexion
PFT	pulmonary function test
P.H., PH, PMH	past history, past medical history
pH	hydrogen-ion concentration
PHO	physician/hospital organizations
PIP	proximal interphalangeal
PiTx	pelvic intermittent traction
PKU	phenylketonuria
pm, p.m.	afternoon
PMH	past medical history
PNF	proprioceptive neuromuscular facilitation
PO	by mouth
POC	plan of care
POD	post-operative day
POE	prone on elbows
polio	poliomyelitis
POMR	problem-oriented medical record
POS	point of service plan
post.	posterior
post	after
post-op	after surgery or operation
PPO	preferred provider organization
pps	pulses per second
PPS	prospective payment system
Pr	problem
PRE	progressive resistive exercise
pre-op	before surgery or operation
prn	whenever necessary, as needed
PROM	passive range of motion
pro time	prothrombin time
prox.	proximal
Prx	prognosis

PSIS	posterior superior iliac spine
PSP	problem, status, plan
PSPG	problem, status, plan, goals
pt	protime
PT	physical therapist, physical therapy
Pt., pt.	patient
PTA	physical therapist assistant, prior to admission
PUW	pick up walker (standard walker)
PVD	peripheral vascular disease
PWB	partial weight-bearing

Q

q̄	every
qd	every day
qh	every hour
qhs	at bedtime
qid	four times a day
qm	every minute
qod	every other day
qt	quart
quad	quadriplegic
quads	quadriceps
qw	once weekly

R

Ⓡ	right
RA	rheumatoid arthritis
RAD	reactive airway disease
RBBB	right bundle branch block
RBC	red blood cells
R.D.	registered dietician
RDS	respiratory distress syndrome
re:	regarding
re-ed	reeducation
REM	rapid eye movement
reps	repetitions
ret.	return
RLE	right lower extremity
RLL	right lower lobe
rm	room
RN	registered nurse
R/O, R.O.	rule out
ROM	range of motion
rot.	rotation
rr	respiratory rate
RROM	resistive range of motion
RT	respiratory therapist
RUE	right upper extremity
RUGs	resource utilization groups
RUL	right upper lobe
Rx	therapy, treatment

S

s̄	without
S	supervision

S:	subjective data
SAH	subarachnoid hemorrhage
SAQ	short arc quadriceps
SB	spontaneously breathing
SBA	standby assist
SCI	spinal cord injury
SDH	subdural hematoma
sec	second(s)
SEC	single-end cane
SGA	small for gestational age
SICU	surgical intensive care unit
SIDS	sudden infant death syndrome
SLB	short leg brace
SLC	short leg cast
SLE	systemic lupus erythematosus
SLP	speech language pathologist
SLR	straight leg raise
SNF	skilled nursing facility
SO	significant other
SOAP	subjective, objective, assessment, plan
SOB	shortness of breath
SOMR	source-oriented medical record
S/P	status post
SPTA	student physical therapist assistant, physical therapist assistant student
SSI	supplemental security income
stat.	immediately, at once
STG	short-term goal
str.	strength
strep	*Streptococcus*
STSG	split-thickness skin graft
sup.	superior
SWD	shortwave diathermy
Sx	symptoms
T	
T	trace muscle strength
T & A	tonsillectomy and adenoidectomy
TB	tuberculosis
TBI	traumatic brain injury
TCO	total contact orthosis
TDD	tentative discharge date
TDP	tentative discharge plan
TDWB	touchdown weight-bearing
T.E.D.S	antiembolitic stockings
temp.	temperature
TENS	transcutaneous electrical nerve stimulation
TF	tube feeding
TFs	transfers
ther. ex.	therapeutic exercise
THR (THA)	total hip replacement (total hip arthroplasty)
TIA	transient ischemic attack
tid	three times a day
TKE	terminal knee extension
TKR (TKA)	total knee replacement (total knee arthroplasty)

TLC	total lung capacity
TMJ	temporomandibular joint
TO	telephone order
tol.	tolerate
trach	tracheostomy
train., trng.	training
TSS	toxic shock syndrome
TT	tilt table
TTWB	toe-touch weight-bearing
TWB	touch weight-bearing
tx	treatment
Tx	traction
TV	tidal volume

U

UA	urinalysis
UCR	usual, customary, and reasonable payment
UE, UEs	upper extremity, upper extremities
UED1	upper extremity diagonal 1
UGI	upper gastrointestinal
UMN	upper motor neuron
UPIN	unique physician identification number
URI	upper respiratory infection
U/S, US	ultrasound
UTI	urinary tract infection
UV	ultraviolet

V

v.c.	verbal cues
VC	vital capacity
VD	venereal disease
vent	ventilator
VO	verbal order
VO$_2$	oxygen consumption
VP	ventricual peritoneal shunt
v.s.	vital signs
VSD	ventricular septal defect
VSU	venous stasis ulcer

W

Ⓦ	wife
w/	with
WB	weight-bearing
WBAT	weight-bearing as tolerated
WBC	white blood cell
WC, w/c	wheelchair
W/cm^2	watts per square centimeter
WBQC	wide-based quad cane
WFL	within functional limits
WHO	World Health Organization
WNL	within normal limits
wk	week
wlp	whirlpool
w/o	without
wt.	weight

X

X	number of times performed
XR	x-ray
xfer (transf)	transfer

Y

YO, y/o	years old
yr	year
YOM	year-old-male

Z

Z	zero

Other Common Symbols:

↔	to and from
↓	down, downward, decrease
↑	up, upward, increase
→	to, progressing forward, approaching
⊥	perpendicular
//	parallel or parallel bars (or // bars)
@, /	per
&	and
'	feet
#	number, pound(s)
Ω	resistance
1X	one time, one person
1°	primary
2°	secondary, secondary to
≈	approximately
+	plus, positive (also abbreviated pos.)
−	minus, negative (negative also abbreviated neg.)
=	equals
≥	greater than
≤	less than
Δ	change
♀	female
♂	male
∴	therefore

Appendix B

Documenting Interventions

SUGGESTED INTERVENTION DOCUMENTATION STYLE

Documenting interventions thoroughly enough so they can be reproduced by another PTA or PT while still keeping the progress note as brief as possible is not easy. The following is a method for providing the appropriate information in a concise format. In this "formula" style for documenting interventions, the information is placed in a continuous line separated by slashes. The information is documented as illustrated here but does not have to be placed in this order: type of intervention/dosage or intensity/treatment area/time/patient position/frequency/purpose.

Examples

Direct contact US/3 MHz/mild heat at (0.5 W/cm^2)/right TMJ/sitting/5 min/to decrease inflammation.

Direct contact US/1 MHz/(1 W/cm^2)/7 min/left middle trapezius & rhomboid/prone/to relax spasm.

Direct contact US/1 MHz/(1.5 W/cm^2)/5 min/Ⓛ shoulder, anterior capsule/sitting/to prepare for stretching.

Induction SWD/large pad/dose III/vigorous heat/L1 to S2/prone/20 min to prepare for stretching.

Intermittent cervical traction/Saunders halter/supine/15 lb/30 sec on, 10 sec off/20 min/to stretch C1–C4 cervical extensors.

Immersion US/1 MHz/right deltoid ligament/sitting/(2 W/cm^2)/10 min/to prepare for stretching.

Static pelvic traction/L4–L5/prone/100 lb/10 min max. or until pain centralizes/to reduce disc bulge.

Ice massage/standard procedure/to numbing response/Ⓡ wrist extensors' tendons at origin/sitting, shoulder abducted 90°, elbow flexed 90° on pillow/after exercise/to minimize inflammatory response.

Hot packs/Ⓡ biceps femoris muscle belly/12 towel layers/prone/20 min/to increase circulation for healing.

Foot whirlpool/110°/decubitus on Ⓛ lateral malleolus/sitting in wheelchair/for mechanical débridement/20 min.

ICP/50 lb/30 sec on, 10 sec off/RUE/elevated 45°/supine/3 hr/to decrease edema.

FES/L anterior tibialis/monopolar/one channel, three leads/two 2-inch square electrodes/origin & insertion/nontreatment electrode under Ⓡ thigh/30 pps/15 min/motor response/pt. semisitting/for muscle reeducation and AAROM.

Appendix C

Dictation Guidelines

In some clinical facilities you will dictate your progress notes instead of writing them. You will dictate or speak into a recording device (such as a small tape recorder or into a telephone), and a medical transcriptionist will listen to the tape and type your note. The typed note will be returned to you to proofread and sign. When learning to dictate progress notes, take the time to write the note first on scrap paper. Then you can read it out loud into the recorder. After you become accustomed to the dictation procedure, you will be able to compose the note and dictate it simultaneously.

GUIDELINES FOR CLEAR DICTATION

Keep in mind that each facility will have guidelines for PTAs. In one clinic, the transcriptionist may be so skilled in typing physical therapy documentation that you will do little more than dictate the content. A medical transcriptionist typically has been trained at a 2-year technical college or community college program. The trained transcriptionist is knowledgeable in medical terminology and punctuation. Another clinic may require that you give specific instructions to the transcriptionist and dictate punctuation. In either case, follow these guidelines for clear dictation:

1. Use proper sentence structure and punctuation, although you can eliminate some wording to keep the note brief.

2. Introduce your dictation by telling the transcriptionist *who you are,* that this is a *progress note,* the *name of your patient,* and the *date of treatment.*

3. Spell out any foreign or unusual names of muscles, treatment techniques, or diagnoses. Clarify <u>abd</u>uct and <u>add</u>uct by spelling out the word.

4. Tell the transcriptionist when you are starting or finishing a note on a particular patient or date, particularly if you are dictating more than one note on a tape.

5. Give your full legal name with your proper abbreviated title (SPTA or PTA) at the end of the dictation.

6. Do not sniff, cough, or chew gum while dictating into the dictaphone.

7. Speak clearly and slowly. Do not mumble.

8. Do not say "uhhh." If you need to collect your thoughts, turn off the tape.

In clinics that require you to give specific instructions to the transcriptionist, follow these additional guidelines:

1. State "operator" just before your instructions to alert the transcriptionist that instructions are to follow, not content.

2. Tell the transcriptionist what letters you want capitalized. However, you can assume the transcriptionist will automatically capitalize the first letter of each sentence. For example: You might say, "Patient's (operator: all in caps) ROM (operator: end of caps) is 0–90 degrees for left knee flexion."

3. Tell the transcriptionist when you are moving to a new heading. For example: "(operator: new heading, all in caps) objective" will come back to you typed "OBJECTIVE."

4. Be aware that you may need to dictate some of the punctuation. For example: You want your note to read, "Transfers: Ⓘ out recliner, on/off toilet, bed after four tries." Your dictation should sound like this: "(Operator: underline capital T) transfers colon independent out recliner comma on slash off toilet comma bed after four tries period."

Appendix D

Guidelines: Physical Therapy Documentation of Patient/Client Management*

BOD G03-05-16-41 (Program 32) [Amended BOD 02-02-16-20; BOD 11-01-06-10; BOD 03-01-16-51; BOD 03-00-22-54; BOD 03-99-14-41; BOD 11-98-19-69; BOD 03-97-27-69; BOD 03-95-23-61; BOD 11-94-33-107; BOD 06-93-09-13; Initial BOD 03-93-21-55] [Guideline]

PREAMBLE

The American Physical Therapy Association (APTA) is committed to meeting the physical therapy needs of society, to meeting the needs and interests of its members, and to developing and improving the art and science of physical therapy, including practice, education, and research. To help meet these responsibilities, the APTA Board of Directors has approved the following guidelines for physical therapy documentation. It is recognized that these guidelines do not reflect all of the unique documentation requirements associated with the many specialty areas within the physical therapy profession. Applicable for both hand written and electronic documentation systems, these guidelines are intended to be used as a foundation for the development of more specific documentation guidelines in clinical areas, while at the same time providing guidance for the physical therapy profession across all practice settings. Documentation may also need to address additional regulatory or payer requirements.

Finally, be aware that these guidelines are intended to address *documentation* of patient/client management, not to describe the provision of physical therapy services. Other APTA documents, including APTA *Standards of Practice for Physical Therapy, Code of Ethics and Guide for Professional Conduct,* and the *Guide to Physical Therapist Practice,* address provision of physical therapy services and patient/client management. The above mentioned documents can be found at the following website: www.apta.org.

APTA POSITION ON DOCUMENTATION

Documentation Authority for Physical Therapy Services

Physical therapy examination, evaluation, diagnosis, prognosis, and intervention shall be documented, dated, and authenticated by the physical therapist who performs the service. Intervention provided by the physical therapist or selected interventions provided by the physical therapist assistant is documented, dated, and authenticated by the physical therapist or, when permissible by law, the physical therapist assistant.

Other notations or flow charts are considered a component of the documented record but do not meet the requirements of documentation in or of themselves. Students in physical therapist or physical therapist assistant programs may document when the record is additionally authenticated by the physical therapist or, when permissible by law, documentation by physical therapist assistant students may be authenticated by a physical therapist assistant.

---

*Adopted by the Board of Directors, APTA March 1993. Amended February 2002, November 2001, March 2000, November 1998, March 1997, November 1994, June 1993, March 1993, June 2003.
From American Physical Therapy Association. (2003). Guidelines for physical therapy documentation. In *Guide to physical therapist practice* (2nd ed., pp. Appendix 695–698). Alexandria, VA: APTA, with permission of the APTA or from the following Web site at www.apta.org.

OPERATIONAL DEFINITIONS

Guidelines: APTA defines a "guideline" as a statement of advice.

Documentation: Any entry into the client record, such as consultation report, initial examination report, progress report, flow sheet/checklist that identifies the care/service provided, reexamination, or summation of care.

Authentication: The process used to verify that an entry is complete, accurate and final. Indications of authentication can include original written signatures and computer "signatures" on secured electronic record systems only.

The following describes the main documentation elements of patient/client management: (1) initial examination/evaluation, (2) visit/encounter, (3) reexamination, and (4) discharge or discontinuation summary.

Initial Examination/ Evaluation

Documentation of the initial encounter is typically called the "initial examination," "initial evaluation," or "initial examination/evaluation." Completion of the initial examination/evaluation is typically completed in one visit but may occur over more than one visit. Documentation elements for the initial examination/evaluation include the following:

Examination: Includes data obtained from the history, systems review, and tests and measures.

Evaluation: Evaluation is a thought process that may not include formal documentation. It may include documentation of the assessment of the data collected in the examination and identification of problems pertinent to patient/client management.

Diagnosis: Indicates the level of impairment and functional limitation determined by the physical therapist. May be indicated by selecting one or more preferred practice patterns from the *Guide to Physical Therapist Practice.*

Prognosis: Provides documentation of the predicted level of improvement that might be attained through intervention and the amount of time required to reach that level. Prognosis is typically not a separate documentation element, but the components are included as part of the plan of care.

Plan of care: Typically stated in general terms, includes goals, interventions planned, proposed frequency and duration, and discharge plan.

Visit/Encounter

Documentation of a visit or encounter, often called a progress note or daily note, documents sequential implementation of the plan of care established by the physical therapist, including changes in patient/client status and variations and progressions of specific interventions used. Also may include specific plans for the next visit or visits.

Reexamination

Documentation of reexamination includes data from repeated or new examination elements and is provided to evaluate progress and to modify or redirect intervention.

Discharge or Discontinuation Summary

Documentation is required following conclusion of the current episode in the physical therapy intervention sequence, to summarize progression toward goals and discharge plans.

I. General Guidelines

A. Documentation is required for every visit/encounter. All documentation must comply with the applicable jurisdictional/regulatory requirements.

1. All handwritten entries shall be made in ink and will include original signatures.

   Electronic entries are made with appropriate security and confidentiality provisions.

2. Charting errors should be corrected by drawing a single line through the error and initialing and dating the chart or through the appropriate mechanism for electronic documentation that clearly indicates that a change was made without deletion of the original record.

3. Identification and Authentication—All documentation must include adequate identification of the patient/client and the physical therapist or physical therapist assistant:

    3.1 The patient's/client's full name and identification number, if applicable, must be included on all official documents.

    3.2 All entries must be dated and authenticated with the provider's full name and appropriate designation.

    3.3 Documentation of examination, evaluation, diagnosis, prognosis, plan of care, and discharge summary must be authenticated by the physical therapist who provided the service.

    3.4 Documentation of intervention in visit/encounter notes must be authenticated by the physical therapist or physical therapist assistant who provided the service.

    3.5 Documentation by physical therapist or physical therapist assistant graduates or other physical therapist and physical therapist assistants pending receipt of an unrestricted license shall be authenticated by a licensed physical therapist, or, when permissible by law, documentation by physical therapist assistant graduates may be authenticated by a physical therapist assistant.

    3.6 Documentation by students (SPT/SPTA) in physical therapist or physical therapist assistant programs must be additionally authenticated by the physical therapist or, when permissible by law, documentation by physical therapist assistant students may be authenticated by a physical therapist assistant.

4. Documentation should include the referral mechanism by which physical therapy services are initiated. Examples include:

    4.1 Self-referral/direct access

    4.2 Request for consultation from another practitioner

5. Documentation should include indication of no shows and cancellations.

II. Initial Patient/Client Management

A. Documentation is required at the onset of each episode of physical therapy care and shall include the elements of examination, evaluation, diagnosis, and prognosis.

B. Documentation of the initial episode of physical therapy care shall include the elements of examination, a comprehensive screening and specific testing process leading to diagnostic classification or, as appropriate, to a referral to another practitioner. The examination has three components: the patient/client history, the systems review, and tests and measures.

1. Documentation of appropriate history.

    1.1 General demographics

    1.2 Social history

    1.3 Employment/work (Job/School/Play)

    1.4 Growth and development

    1.5 Living environment

    1.6 General health status (self-report, family report, caregiver report)

    1.7 Social/health habits (past and current)

    1.8 Family history

    1.9 Medical/surgical history

    1.10 Current condition(s)/Chief complaint(s)

    1.11 Functional status and activity level

    1.12 Medications

    1.13 Other clinical tests

2. Documentation of systems review

    2.1 Documentation of physiologic and anatomical status to include the following systems.

        2.1.1 **Cardiovascular/pulmonary**

            2.1.1.1 Blood pressure

            2.1.1.2 Edema

2.1.1.3 Heart rate

2.1.1.4 Respiratory rate

2.1.2 **Integumentary**

2.1.2.1 Presence of scar formation

2.1.2.2 Skin color

2.1.2.3 Skin integrity

2.1.3 **Musculoskeletal**

2.1.3.1 Gross range of motion

2.1.3.2 Gross strength

2.1.3.3 Gross symmetry

2.1.3.4 Height

2.1.3.5 Weight

2.1.4 **Neuromuscular**

2.1.4.1 Gross coordinated movement (e.g., balance, locomotion, transfers, and transitions)

2.2 Documentation of systems review may also address communication ability, affect, cognition, language, and learning style:

2.2.1 Ability to make needs known

2.2.2 Consciousness

2.2.3 Orientation (person, place, time)

2.2.4 Expected emotional/behavioral responses

2.2.5 Learning preferences

3. Documentation of selection and administration of appropriate tests and measures to determine patient/client status in a number of areas and documentation of findings. The following is a list of the areas to be addressing the documented examination and evaluation, including illustrative tests and measures for each area:

3.1 *Aerobic capacity/endurance*

Examples of examination findings include:

3.1.1 Aerobic capacity during functional activities

3.1.2 Aerobic capacity during standardized exercise test protocols

3.1.3 Cardiovascular signs and symptoms in response to increased oxygen demand with exercise or activity

3.1.4 Pulmonary signs and symptoms in response to increased oxygen demand with exercise or activity

3.2 *Anthropometric characteristics*

Examples of examination findings include:

3.2.1 Body composition

3.2.2 Body dimensions

3.2.3 Edema

3.3 *Arousal, attention, and cognition*

Examples of examination findings include:

3.3.1 Arousal and attention

3.3.2 Cognition

3.3.3 Communication

3.3.4 Consciousness

3.3.5 Motivation

3.3.6 Orientation to time, person, place, and situation

3.3.7 Recall

3.4 *Assistive and adaptive devices*

Examples of examination findings include:

3.4.1 Assistive or adaptive devices and equipment use during functional activities

3.4.2 Components, alignment, fit, and ability to care for the assistive or adaptive devices and equipment

3.4.3 Remediation of impairments, functional limitations, or disabilities with use of assistive or adaptive devices and equipment

3.4.4 Safety during use of assistive or adaptive devices and equipment

3.5 *Circulation (arterial, venous, lymphatic)*
Examples of examination findings include:
3.5.1 Cardiovascular signs
3.5.2 Cardiovascular symptoms
3.5.3 Physiological responses to position change

3.6 *Cranial and peripheral nerve integrity*
Examples of examination findings include:
3.6.1 Electrophysiological integrity
3.6.2 Motor distribution of the cranial nerves
3.6.3 Motor distribution of the peripheral nerves
3.6.4 Response to neural provocation
3.6.5 Response to stimuli, including auditory, gustatory, olfactory, pharyngeal, vestibular, and visual
3.6.6 Sensory distribution of the cranial nerves
3.6.7 Sensory distribution of the peripheral nerves

3.7 *Environmental, home, and work (job/school/play) barriers*
Examples of examination findings include:
3.7.1 Current and potential barriers
3.7.2 Physical space and environment

3.8 *Ergonomics and body mechanics*
Examples of examination findings for *ergonomics* include:
3.8.1 Dexterity and coordination during work
3.8.2 Functional capacity and performance during work actions, tasks, or activities
3.8.3 Safety in work environments
3.8.4 Specific work conditions or activities
3.8.5 Tools, devices, equipment, and work-stations related to work actions, tasks, or activities
Examples of examination findings for *body mechanics* include:
3.8.6 Body mechanics during self-care, home management, work, community, or leisure actions, tasks, or activities

3.9 *Gait, locomotion, and balance*
Examples of examination findings include:
3.9.1 Balance during functional activities with or without the use of assistive, adaptive, orthotic, protection, supportive, or prosthetic devices or equipment
3.9.2 Balance (dynamic and static) with or without the use of assistive, adaptive, orthotic, protective, supportive, or prosthetic devices or equipment
3.9.3 Gait and locomotion during functional activities with or without the use of assistive, adaptive, orthotic, protective, supportive, or prosthetic devices or equipment
3.9.4 Gait and locomotion with or without the use of assistive, adaptive, orthotic, protective, supportive, or prosthetic devices or equipment
3.9.5 Safety during gait, locomotion, and balance

3.10 *Integumentary integrity*
Examples of examination findings include:
3.10.1 Associated skin:
3.10.1.1 Activities, positioning, and postures that produce or relieve trauma to the skin
3.10.1.2 Assistive, adaptive, orthotic, protective, supportive, or prosthetic devices and equipment that may produce or relieve trauma to the skin
3.10.1.3 Skin characteristics

3.10.2 Wound:

    3.10.2.1 Activities, positioning, and postures that aggravate the wound or scar or that produce or relieve trauma

    3.10.2.2 Burn

    3.10.2.3 Signs of infection

    3.10.2.4 Wound characteristics

    3.10.2.5 Wound scar tissue characteristics

3.11 *Joint integrity and mobility*

Examples of examination findings include:

3.11.1 Joint integrity and mobility

3.11.2 Joint play movements

3.11.3 Specific body parts

3.12 *Motor function*

Examples of examination findings include:

3.12.1 Dexterity, coordination, and agility

3.12.2 Electrophysiological integrity

3.12.3 Hand function

3.12.4 Initiation, modification, and control of movement patterns and voluntary postures

3.13 *Muscle performance*

Examples of examination findings include:

3.13.1 Electrophysiological integrity

3.13.2 Muscle strength, power, and endurance

3.13.3 Muscle strength, power, and endurance during functional activities

3.13.4 Muscle tension

3.14 *Neuromotor development and sensory integration*

Examples of examination findings include:

3.14.1 Acquisition and evolution of motor skills

3.14.2 Oral motor function, phonation, and speech production

3.14.3 Sensorimotor integration

3.15 *Orthotic, protective, and supportive devices*

Examples of examination findings include:

3.15.1 Components, alignment, fit, and ability to care for the orthotic, protective, and supportive devices and equipment

3.15.2 Orthotic, protective, and supportive devices and equipment use during functional activities

3.15.3 Remediation of impairments, functional limitations, or disabilities with use of orthotic, protective, and supportive devices and equipment

3.15.4 Safety during use of orthotic, protective, and supportive devices and equipment

3.16 *Pain*

Examples of examination findings include:

3.16.1 Pain, soreness, and nocioception

3.16.2 Pain in specific body parts

3.17 *Posture*

Examples of examination findings include:

3.17.1 Postural alignment and position (dynamic)

3.17.2 Postural alignment and position (static)

3.17.3 Specific body parts

3.18 *Prosthetic requirements*

Examples of examination findings include:

3.18.1 Components, alignment, fit, and ability to care for prosthetic device

3.18.2 Prosthetic device use during functional activities

            3.18.3 Remediation of impairments, functional limitations, or disabilities with use of the prosthetic device

            3.18.4 Residual limb or adjacent segment

            3.18.5 Safety during use of the prosthetic device

       3.19 *Range of motion (including muscle length)*

       Examples of examination findings include:

            3.19.1 Functional ROM

            3.19.2 Joint active and passive movement

            3.19.3 Muscle length, soft tissue extensibility, and flexibility

       3.20 *Reflex integrity*

       Examples of examination findings include:

            3.20.1 Deep reflexes

            3.20.2 Electrophysiological integrity

            3.20.3 Postural reflexes and reactions, including righting, equilibrium, and protective reactions

            3.20.4 Primitive reflexes and reactions

            3.20.5 Resistance to passive stretch

            3.20.6 Superficial reflexes and reactions

       3.21 *Self-care and home management (including activities of daily living and instrumental activities of daily living)*

       Examples of examination findings include:

            3.21.1 Ability to gain access to home environments

            3.21.2 Ability to perform self-care and home management activities with or without assistive, adaptive, orthotic, protective, supportive, or prosthetic devices and equipment

            3.21.3 Safety in self-care and home management activities and environments

       3.22 *Sensory integrity*

       Examples of examination findings include:

            3.22.1 Combined/cortical sensations

            3.22.2 Deep sensations

            3.22.3 Electrophysiological integrity

       3.23 *Ventilation and respiration*

       Examples of examination findings include:

            3.23.1 Pulmonary signs of respiration/gas exchange

            3.23.2 Pulmonary signs of ventilatory function

            3.23.3 Pulmonary symptoms

       3.24 *Work (job/school/play), community, and leisure integration or reintegration (including instrumental activities of daily living)*

       Examples of examination findings include:

            3.24.1 Ability to assume or resume work (job/school/play), community, and leisure activities with or without assistive, adaptive, orthotic, protective, supportive, or prosthetic devices and equipment

            3.24.2 Ability to gain access to work (job/school/play), community, and leisure environments

            3.24.3 Safety in work (job/school/play), community, and leisure activities and environments

C. Documentation of evaluation (a dynamic process in which the physical therapist makes clinical judgments based on data gathered during the examination).

D. Documentation of diagnosis, a label that identifies the impact of the condition on function at the level of the system, especially the movement system, and at the level of the whole person in terms that can guide the prognosis, the plan of care, and intervention strategies.

E. Documentation of prognosis (determination of the level of optimal improvement that might be attained through intervention and the amount of time required to reach that level. Documentation shall include goals, outcomes, and plan of care).

1. Patient/client (and family members and significant others, if appropriate) is involved in establishing goals and outcomes.
2. All goals and outcomes are stated in measurable terms.
3. Goals and outcomes are related to impairments, functional limitation, and disabilities and the changes in health, wellness, and fitness needs identified in the examination.
4. The plan of care:
   4.1 Is based on the examination, evaluation, diagnosis, and prognosis.
   4.2 Identifies goals and outcomes of all proposed interventions.
   4.3 Describes the proposed interventions taking into consideration the expectations of the patient/client and others as appropriate.
   4.4 Includes frequency and duration of all proposed interventions to achieve the anticipated goals and expected outcomes.
   4.5 Involves appropriate coordination and communication of care with other professionals/services.
   4.6 Includes plan for discharge.
F. Authentication by and appropriate designation of the physical therapist.

III. Documentation of the Continuation of Care

A. Documentation of intervention or services provided and current patient/client status.
   1. Documentation is required for every visit/encounter.
      1.1 Authentication and appropriate designation of the physical therapist or the physical therapist assistant providing the service under the direction and supervision of a physical therapist.
   2. Documentation of each visit/encounter shall include the following elements:
      2.1 Patient/client self-report (as appropriate).
      2.2 Identification of specific interventions provided, including frequency, intensity, and duration as appropriate.
         Examples include:
         2.2.1 Knee extension, 3 sets, 10 repetitions, 10-lb weight.
         2.2.2 Transfer training bed to chair with sliding board.
      2.3 Equipment provided.
      2.4 Changes in patient/client status as they relate to the plan of care.
      2.5 Adverse reaction to interventions, if any.
      2.6 Factors that modify frequency or intensity of intervention and progression toward anticipated goals, including patient/client adherence to patient/client-related instructions.
      2.7 Communication/consultation with providers/patient/client/family/significant other.
B. Documentation of reexamination
   1. Documentation of reexamination is provided as appropriate to evaluate progress and to modify or redirect intervention.
   2. Documentation of reexamination should include the following elements:
      2.1 Documentation of selected components of examination to update patient's/client's status.
      2.2 Interpretation of findings and, when indicated, revision of goals and outcomes.
      2.3 When indicated, revision of plan of care as directly correlated with goals and outcomes as documented.
      2.4 Authentication by an appropriate designation of the physical therapist.

IV. Documentation of Summation of Episode of Care

A. Documentation is required following conclusion of the current episode in the physical therapy intervention sequence.

B. Documentation of the summation of the episode of care shall include the following elements:

1. Criteria for termination of services:

   Examples of discharge include:

   1.1 Anticipated goals and expected outcomes have been achieved.

   Examples of discontinuation include:

   1.2 Patient/client, caregiver, or legal guardian declines to continue intervention.

   1.3 Patient/client is unable to continue to progress toward anticipated goals due to medical or psychosocial complications or because financial/insurance resources have been expended.

   1.4 Physical therapist determines that the patient/client will no longer benefit from physical therapy.

2. Current physical/functional status.

3. Degree of goals and outcomes achieved and reasons for goals and outcomes not being achieved.

4. Discharge or discontinuation plan that includes written and verbal communication related to the patient's/client's continuing care.

   Examples include:

   4.1 Home program

   4.2 Referrals for additional services

   4.3 Recommendations for follow-up physical therapy care

   4.4 Family and caregiver training

   4.5 Equipment provided

5. Authentication by and appropriate designation of the physical therapist.

REFERENCES

1. *Direction and Supervision of the Physical Therapist Assistant* (HOD 06-00-16-27) www.apta.org.
2. *Comprehensive Accreditation Manual for Hospitals.* Oakbrook Terrace, Ill: Joint Commission on the Accreditation of Healthcare Organizations; 1996.
3. *Glossary of Terms Related to Information Security.* Schaumburg, Ill: Computer-based Patient Record Institute; 1996.
4. *Guidelines for Establishing Information Security Policies at Organizations Using Computer-based Patient Records.* Schaumburg, Ill: Computer-based Patient Record Institute; 1995.
5. *Current Procedural Terminology.* Chicago, Ill: American Medical Association (AMA); 2000.
6. *Coding and Payment Guide for the Physical Therapist.* Washington, DC: St. Anthony's Publishing; 2000.
7. Healthcare Financing Administration (HCFA); Minimal Data Set (MDS) Regulations, HCFA/AMA Documentation Guidelines, Home Health Regulations. Available at: www.hcfa.gov.
8. State Practice Acts. Available at: www.fsbpt.org.

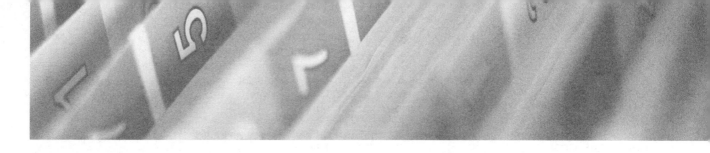

INDEX

Page numbers followed by a "b" indicate a box; page numbers followed by an "f" indicate a figure; page numbers followed by a "t" indicate a table.

DISCARD

CERRO'S COLLEGE LIBRARY
Menlo Park, California